Essentials of Delirium

Essentials of Delirium

Everything You Really Need to Know for Working in Delirium Care

Dr Shibley Rahman

Forewords by Prof. Sharon Inouye
and Prof. Alasdair MacLullich

Afterwords by Dr Daniel Davis and Dr Amit Arora

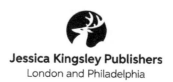

Jessica Kingsley Publishers
London and Philadelphia

Personal account on pp.170–1 reproduced with kind permission of Mark Hudson.
Figure 1.1 reproduced with kind permission of Prof. Alasdair MacLullich.
Figure 1.2 reproduced with kind permission of Prof. Alasdair MacLullich.
Figure 4AT not to be reproduced without permission.
Figure 2.1 reproduced with kind permission of Prof. Sharon Inouye. Confusion Assessment Method. Copyright 2003, Hospital Elder Life Program, LLC. Not to be reproduced without permission. No responsibility is assumed by the AGS or the Hospital Elder Life Program, LLC for any injury and/or damage to persons or property arising out of the application of any of the content at help.agscocare.org.
Figure 9.1 reproduced with kind permission of Prof. Alasdair MacLullich.

First published in 2020
by Jessica Kingsley Publishers
73 Collier Street
London N1 9BE, UK

www.jkp.com

Library of Congress Cataloging in Publication Data
A CIP catalog record for this book is available from the Library of Congress

British Library Cataloguing in Publication Data
A CIP catalogue record for this book is available from the British Library

ISBN 978 1 78592 673 0
eISBN 978 1 78592 674 7

Printed and bound in Great Britain

To my mum.

Contents

Preface

It's been a pleasure to write this book purely for personal reasons.

This book is not about managing a condition. It is about caring for a person. This is challenging – but the potential rewards are huge.

Whatever your view of cognitive neuropsychology, one based on the modularity of mind or one based on distributed neuronal networks, delirium represents perhaps the ultimate challenge.

As I know from my own experience, watching a loved one flip in and out of 'delirium' is profoundly shocking. There was a time when the attitude that 'this is just what happens to older people' was seen as a legitimate response to delirium. Thankfully, times have changed.

Delirium is a cause of major emotional distress to those around, including staff. It could also lead your loved one never to return home after a hospital admission, but instead lead to a fast transfer to a nursing home.

It could perhaps lead to an accelerated decline in cognitive function.

Delirium has a huge, if largely unmeasured, financial impact, including indirect costs and opportunity cost.

It seems rather perplexing that all the doctors on a ward round might genuinely seem unperturbed by a patient in deep sleep, hard to rouse at 11am in a busy, noisy ward, with the curtains wide open. In response to a basic enquiry from a relative, who has fought hard to be on the ward during 'visiting hours', a doctor might not actually be able to explain what has caused this rapid change in personality and behaviour, or when this horror of the delirium experience will finally be over.

Delirium can happen in any care setting, including at home. We need anyone involved in care, especially of those at risk, including people with dementia, to be able to spot it (Chapter 1: Delirium awareness). On suspecting it, we need delirium to be identified, diagnosed and managed appropriately (Chapter 2: Delirium identification, assessment and diagnosis). Some individuals are particularly at risk of dementia (Chapter 3: Delirium risk reduction and prevention), and it's worth knowing how one might minimise the chances of developing dementia.

For that period of time when a person is experiencing a delirium, that person takes a temporary diversion from his own life course. It's as if his sense of personhood has been 'suspended'. But it's worth thinking about the significant effects of suspending a patient's identity as a person. The full force of this argument would be to strip him of dignity and of an entitlement to other human rights. It is shocking that relatively little attention has been given to addressing how to optimise the conditions for person-centred care, but this should be a goal of high-quality care (Chapter 4: Person-centred delirium care).

Communication is not only essential between the person experiencing delirium and all those providing care, but is also essential between all members of an interprofessional team for effective teamwork (Chapter 5: Communication, interaction and behaviour in delirium care). Even if a person with delirium himself is uncommunicative, the promotion of health and wellbeing – for example, early mobilisation and good nutrition and hydration – are critical (Chapter 6: Health and wellbeing in delirium).

There is an impressive army of interventions in delirium, including non-pharmacological and pharmacological approaches (Chapter 7: Interventions in delirium care). Given that we do not understand the precise neuroscience behind delirium, work in this space has been surprisingly successful. But there is now robust recognition that patients can have a range of outcomes after delirium (Chapter 8: Outcomes after delirium episodes), which means that prompt recognition and management of delirium is a moral imperative as well as a legal one from the perspective of patient safety. A person with delirium might have long-lasting psychological effects of the delirium episode, and the power of stories of survivors of delirium cannot be underestimated (Chapter 9: The delirium experience). Enabling and protecting a person while experiencing delirium must be achieved somehow, and all persons involved in high-quality delirium care must understand the current legal and ethical issues. Only this way can one understand how decisions may be made in care, and also why objections are raised against restraints and inappropriate chemical medication (Chapter 10: Law, ethics and safeguarding in delirium care). Knowing when delirium is reversible, appreciating what to do when somebody with delirium is in his last days, and understanding the scope of services is important for anyone with an interest in palliative and end-of-life care in delirium (Chapter 11: Palliative and end-of-life care, and delirium).

Beneficial improvements in providing high-quality care through quality improvement are easier to achieve when interested parties are involved in, rather than the recipients of, change (Chapter 12: Evidence-based medicine and quality improvement). Educational initiatives, whether developments in the undergraduate curriculum or innovations in service provision such as the use of simulations or e-learning, continue to ensure that a well-trained workforce can recognise and do something about delirium (Chapter 13: Educational initiatives).

Delirium matters

Delirium is a major unmet need in modern acute hospitals. As the population ages, it will become more common. Education, training and overall quality improvement are effective in improving the care of delirium.

Three important 'action points' are:

1. Identify a member of staff (e.g. a doctor or nurse with specialist skills in the care of older people) to take the lead in education and care.

2. Measure rates of delirium identification.

3. Incorporate delirium care into corporate and quality practices.

A multidisciplinary approach enables high-quality care and improves patient outcomes.

Reducing variation in care, involving families and optimising the environment are all important elements in managing delirium. That the single delirium event can have huge repercussions has been a rude awakening, but a necessary one, I feel.

A word of warning

You'll find some topics repeated in the text, discussed in different ways, as the book progresses. This is entirely deliberate on my part, to try to emphasise what are important and overlooked messages.

Nothing in this book should be taken as professional legal or clinical advice.

And a word of thanks

I am grateful to Professor Alasdair MacLullich (Edinburgh) and Professor Sharon Inouye (Harvard) for their Forewords, and to Dr Daniel Davis (London) and Dr Amit Arora (Stoke-on-Trent) for their Afterwords. I am also especially grateful to Mark Hudson for sharing an account of his 'delirium experience' in Chapter 9. I would like to thank Tor Butler-Cole QC for a discussion of the current legislation on deprivation of liberty. I'm further grateful to the organisers of the Royal College of Physicians of Edinburgh/European Delirium Association meeting on delirium in Edinburgh in 2019, for a stimulating and wide-ranging meeting which has influenced the content and shape of this book.

Finally, I'd like to thank my mum for teaching me all the really important stuff about delirium. I will always be eternally grateful.

Dr Shibley Rahman PhD (Cantab) MRCP (UK) LLM MBA
London, November 2019

Foreword

Prof. Sharon Inouye

Delirium, defined as an acute disorder of attention and cognition, is a common, life-threatening, and potentially preventable clinical syndrome in older persons. Commonly occurring following acute illness, surgery, or hospitalization, the development of delirium often initiates a cascade of events culminating in increased morbidity and mortality, loss of independence, need for institutionalization, tremendous caregiver burden, and high healthcare costs. Importantly, steadily mounting evidence suggests that delirium is associated with long-term cognitive decline, including incident or accelerated dementia. In the United States, delirium affects over 2.6 million older adults per year, with costs of more than $164 billion per year in healthcare expenditures attributable to delirium. Comparable rates are cited in the European Union, with estimates of over $182 billion per year attributable to delirium in 18 European countries combined.

Given its adverse impact on functioning and quality of life with potentially permanent sequelae, delirium holds tremendous societal implications for the individual, family, community, and healthcare systems. In fact, delirium is increasingly recognized as a public health priority. Clearly, delirium fulfils the defining criteria of a public health condition:[1] (1) a large burden of disease; (2) disproportionately affects certain subgroups, such as older, vulnerable, chronically ill adults; (3) epidemic prone – the 'silent epidemic' of unrecognised delirium; and (4) effective prevention strategies demonstrated, such as the Hospital Elder Life Program (HELP). Large-scale public education campaigns about delirium are being launched, such as by the Global Brain Health Initiative of the American Association of Retired Persons (AARP), the Age-Friendly Hospital movement by the Institute for Healthcare Improvement, and the International Drive to Illuminate

Delirium (IDID) by *Alzheimer's & Dementia: The Journal of the Alzheimer's Association.*

This book by Dr Shibley Rahman, intended for healthcare professionals, families, caregivers, and all other interested parties, represents a singular and essential addition to the literature about delirium. The book springs from Dr Rahman's personal experiences as a caregiver for his mother, suffering with dementia, who has experienced multiple episodes of delirium. Thus, the book is a labor of love, to educate caregivers about this important topic and to share his knowledge and experience. His passion and caring show on each page; this is a well-researched and comprehensive guide to delirium – focused on care at the bedside.

In healthcare, since knowledge is our main weapon, this book will serve valiantly in our fight against delirium. The problem is common, serious, often devastating, and will touch the lives of millions of families worldwide. Read on; we have many valuable lessons to learn from Dr Rahman.

Prof. Sharon Inouye, MD, MPH
Harvard, November 2019

Endnote

1   World Health Organization (2007) *Scoping Paper: Priority Public Health Conditions.* Geneva: WHO. Accessed on 13/12/2019 at www.who.int/social_determinants/resources/pphc_scoping_paper.pdf.

Foreword

Prof. Alasdair MacLullich

Delirium is in many ways an odd condition in modern medical practice. It has been recognised for millennia, and is present in around one in six people in hospital. It can cause severe distress in people with the condition as well as their loved ones. Dr Rahman's account in this book of his own experience of caring for his mother with delirium persuasively illustrates this.

In addition to the manifest suffering that delirium causes, studies show that delirium predicts many other bad outcomes and that its economic costs are staggering. Yet in most healthcare settings most people with delirium still do not receive a diagnosis. Partly as a result, most receive poor or limited treatment. Evidence-based methods of reducing the risk of delirium in hospitalised people, achieved mainly by avoiding iatrogenic harms such as dehydration, are not generally implemented. Additionally, families are mostly not informed of the diagnosis, adding hugely to the stress caused by witnessing the illness itself.

The body of research on delirium has recently been growing rapidly but is still disproportionately small. For example, the 2019 Scottish Intercollegiate Guidelines Network (SIGN) Guidelines[1] on delirium found only three randomised control trials of systematic multicomponent delirium treatment. This form of treatment is the mainstay of delirium treatment in clinical practice.

Another peculiarity of the field is that despite the fact that staff in acute settings see delirium day to day, they are mostly ill-trained in delirium care. The main cause of this is that the profile of delirium in undergraduate and postgraduate training remains worryingly low: recent studies show that healthcare students often receive no or minimal education on delirium.

But perhaps the most striking indicator of the odd position of delirium is that books focused on delirium are rare. Only a handful have been published. This is a major obstacle to the mainstreaming of delirium because review articles are relatively inaccessible to practitioners, and because they cannot provide the comprehensiveness and depth of a book. This text is a unique contribution and fills a major gap. Its uncompromising emphasis on the experience of patients is extremely welcome. Yet it also provides a general overview of delirium care at the bedside as well as the necessary organisational, educational and policy advances that we need to improve outcomes for people with delirium. *Essentials of Delirium* should become a go-to text for frontline healthcare workers, policy-makers and others who seek a readable, clear and practice-orientated account of delirium.

Prof. Alasdair MacLullich
Edinburgh, November 2019

Endnote

1   Health Improvement Scotland (2019) *SIGN 157: Risk Reduction and Management of Delirium. A National Clinical Guideline.* Accessed on 28/11/2019 at www.sign.ac.uk/assets/sign157.pdf.

1

Delirium awareness

LEARNING OBJECTIVES

To provide an overview of the importance of detection and management of delirium, and to consider 'barriers' to good-quality person-centred delirium care. You will be introduced to the notion of simple 'screening tests', and also to the potential identification of distinct delirium syndromes.

What do we do?

Delirium is a 'top-down' phenotype.

Delirium can be prevented and treated:[1] use the **3Rs** – **R**isk assess (possible causes), **R**ecognise (fluctuation in cognition or behaviour) and **R**eact (manage appropriately).

This has also been phrased as 'Spot it – Treat it – Stop it'.

We have to focus on the aetiology initially.

Ask the question: Is he/she different *today*?

Why is delirium important?

Delirium is a common and serious condition among the elderly, particularly in hospitalised patients, affecting up to 30% of this patient population.[2] More recent studies report a prevalence of delirium of 10–31% on admission and an incidence of 3–29% during hospitalisation.[3]

Delirium has been known of since ancient times. Yet there is much evidence that delirium represents a largely unrecognised condition affecting older people within contemporary healthcare internationally. The third-century Greek philosopher Celsus was reportedly the first to use the word 'delirium' to describe mental disorders. The Latin *delirare* means 'to be off the track' or 'to go wrong'.

A statement from ten Societies in 2020 has suggested that the term 'acute encephalopathy' should refer to a rapidly developing (over less than four weeks, but usually within hours to a few days) pathobiological process in the brain.[4] This acute encephalopathy can lead to a clinical presentation of subsyndromal delirium, delirium, or in case of a severely decreased level of consciousness, coma; all representing a change from baseline cognitive status.

The onset of delirium is sudden, and often very shocking to onlookers. There are reasons for thinking of delirium as the AKI ('acute kidney injury') of the brain. Reasons include:

- Both AKI and delirium can have very sudden onset.

- Chronic counterparts exist, e.g. chronic kidney disease and dementia.

- Both AKI and delirium can be easily precipitated if the organs concerned have low 'resilience' or 'reserve'.

- Both can be managed by withdrawal of a precipitant or treatment of a cause.

- They might be triggered by similar causes, e.g. constipation, infection, change in medication, polypharmacy.

- Both AKI and delirium, if missed, can lead to terrible consequences in morbidity and mortality.

The ubiquitous nature of delirium possibly means that no single field of medicine has taken true clinical and research responsibility or 'ownership' for it as an entity. This has led to some difficulties in agreeing on a consensus, especially about which clinicians are the most suitable to get involved. The most profound danger is that healthcare providers can sometimes view older patients as unable to benefit from the various measures that would be used in younger adults. However, most people believe that delirium is 'everybody's business', and professionals of different backgrounds have valid complementary skills to contribute.

The introduction to the celebrated article 'Delirium, a syndrome of cerebral insufficiency'[5] by Engel and Romano (1959) is still chilling:

It is a curious fact that while most physicians have a strong view toward an organic etiology of mental disturbances, at the same time they seem to have little interest in, and, indeed, often overlook delirium, the one mental disorder present known to be a derangement of cerebral metabolism.

Delirium is known by several terms, some still in use in clinical practice. These terms include 'acute brain failure', 'acute confusional state', 'acute confusion', 'acute on chronic confusion' and 'acute encephalopathy'.

The term 'delirium' rather than the somewhat ill-defined alternatives is more commonly used, but this common usage can promote diagnostic rates, standardisation of care and easier communication between healthcare professionals and crucially with patients and carers. Most significantly, it enables a sense of interprofessional interoperability. The use of 'delirium' as an umbrella term is important in engaging and educating colleagues throughout the healthcare ecosystem.

Only in 1980, with the publication of the third edition of the American Psychiatric Association's *Diagnostic and Statistical Manual* (DSM-III) were standardised diagnostic criteria established.

But some feel that the time is now right to change the name of the disorder from delirium to another name which could enhance the credibility and detract from ill-formed ideas, beliefs and prejudices about delirium.

The delirium episode is associated with increased morbidity and mortality. The duration of hospital stay increases, the risk of developing dementia increases, and the risks of morbidity and mortality increase. Furthermore, patients who experience an episode of delirium may subsequently suffer loss of function and increased dependence. As delirium is to a large degree a preventable syndrome, this is quite unacceptable.

You can, however, make a difference if you recognise delirium early and escalate it.

Although delirium is usually caused by alterations in physiological function, its manifestations are almost always behavioural, cognitive, motor, affective or motivational, and thus the recognition of this multifaceted syndrome can be difficult. It often starts suddenly and usually lifts when the root cause gets better (but there can be a lag). It can be intensely distressing and frightening – not only for the person who is unwell, but also for those around him or her.

Any person can get delirium, but it is more common when a person is older, is frail, has a pre-existing cognitive or sensory impairment or is simply very ill.

Sadly, a majority of delirium episodes remain missed entirely or misdiagnosed by clinical teams. Across all jurisdictions, professional regulatory codes require that clinicians keep their knowledge up to date, assess patients' needs and propose management options to the best of their abilities, based on the best evidence available and best practice. There is also a requirement for clinicians to share with people, their families and their carers, as far as the current law allows, the information they want or need to know about their health, care and ongoing treatment sensitively and in a way they can understand.

Flaws in delirium care

Tackling delirium is a collective endeavour.

Delirium is actually a very common finding in the acute hospital setting.[6] It is also now recognised that healthcare systems and services frequently have attributes that unintentionally stimulate or aggravate delirium.

Patient safety results from the interaction of multiple influences in complex and unpredictable healthcare environments. A plethora of attempts have been made to improve safety and reduce harm in delirium care, using different interventions and quality improvement initiatives. Delirium can also be regarded as the 'canary in the mineshaft' of the global quality of care in hospitals and also in long-term care settings when the low level of technological equipment gives a particularly important role to direct clinical observation.

In the UK, there is an increasing consensus that staff working within the acute hospital setting lack the necessary skills and knowledge to effectively manage patients with delirium. Clinical staff might detect different delirium features, which has clear implications for staff education and training. For example, it is sometimes said that nursing staff notice attentional and psychotic phenomena, whereas medical staff tend to detect delirium in the presence of mnemonic problems. General hospitals can have poorly developed care systems that are not yet fully aligned to the needs of this important yet vulnerable group. Optimal management of delirium primarily depends on reducing modifiable risk factors and detecting 'high-risk' cases early.

Unfortunately, stigma might also be a barrier against delirium being treated as a priority. Stigma is conceptualised as a complex social process co-occurring with labelling, stereotyping, under-valuation and 'otherness'. The field of delirium, arguably, faces innumerable challenges in terms of continued stigma and funding shortfalls for clinical care and research.[7] Stigma arises out of normal human cognitive processes that contribute to self-image. Since power dynamics are essential to the social production of stigma, with the label of 'stigmatised person' being likely given by those with power, it is not surprising that stigmatisation occurs on multiple levels for a diverse range of physical and mental conditions. Delirium is at the cusp of both mental and physical illbeing. Addressing such obstructive attitudes to care might facilitate the detection of delirium. We need more advanced exploration about 'mimetic' learning to see how informal attitudes can be changed to improve quality of care.[8]

There is growing evidence of persistent obstacles in delirium care across Europe including (a) attitude, culture and language; (b) knowledge, skills and education; (c) organisation. However, pursuing educational initiatives is time-consuming and labour-intensive.[9]

An overall approach to the patient with delirium

A helpful way of thinking about key aspects of delirium care is provided by MacLullich, which he calls the **Delirium 8** (Figure 1.1).

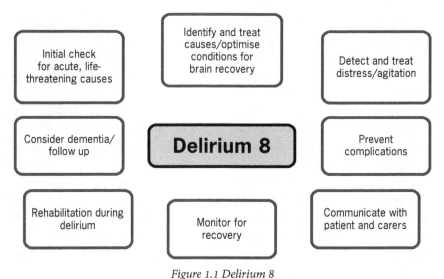

Figure 1.1 Delirium 8

Reproduced by kind permission of Prof. Alasdair MacLullich.

Prof. Alasdair MacLullich is Professor of Geriatric Medicine at the University of Edinburgh, but is best known perhaps for his ground-breaking work in coming up with ways to understand and detect delirium, share the importance of this with colleagues, and distinguish patients with delirium from those with dementia.

Detecting delirium

Delirium detection should ideally be undertaken at the earliest opportunity. It might conceivably be done by an unpaid family carer who notices subtle changes in a relative's personality, cognition and behaviour, even prior to a hospital admission.

Because delirium is so common, all healthcare staff having contact with acutely unwell patients need to assume responsibility for detecting and treating it, as well as aiming to reduce the risk of delirium occurring in the first place. Those working in the long-term care environment should be able to recognise delirium, mitigate against risk and monitor those in their care to resolve delirium. This includes care at home by unpaid family carers. Assessment and knowledge of the usual level of cognitive functioning and behaviour of patients are vital for the early recognition and investigation of delirium, and are crucial to their optimal management and healthcare outcomes across all healthcare systems.

There has been a shift towards recognising delirium as a distinct entity requiring study in its own right rather than being simply a 'secondary' or 'minor' issue. Where delirium is detected, the diagnosis of delirium should be clearly documented to aid transfers of care (e.g. handover notes, referral and discharge letters). 'Delirium awareness' has thankfully resulted in greater appreciation of the variety of the syndrome's symptoms and the development of accurate screening tools that can be readily applied in routine clinical practice. There is no disagreement about the need to involve as many people as possible in good delirium care.

This can happen at all stages of any care pathway. Prompt recognition and identification of delirium upon admission by emergency services have the potential to improve patient outcomes and provide major cost savings to the hospital. Many delirium tools have already been developed, but they differ in terms of intended use, training requirements, properties and suitability for patients in various diverse care settings.

A formal assessment and diagnosis must be made by a suitably trained clinician whenever patients with probable delirium are identified. Where screening is done by nurses, but diagnosis and investigation is done by doctors, systems need to be in place to ensure that information on those screening positive is shared easily. This could be facilitated by modern electronic systems.

It is important to be aware that delirium may still occur in the absence of a positive test result because the condition fluctuates. Healthcare staff should not rely on the result of a single assessment during hospital admission. Possible reasons for the low sensitivity in the detection of delirium include an insensitivity to hypoactive delirium, the complexity or failure to administer tools to assess mental status, and the fact that physicians are usually not trained to use or are not comfortable in using these tools. Many patients with delirium can be too drowsy or agitated to respond to cognitive tests.[10]

Barriers exist to screening for delirium. One well-described barrier is a 'knowledge deficit' among clinicians. If delirium is missed by clinicians, it cannot possibly be managed well. Addressing this is considered in greater detail in Chapter 13.

Some well-known screening tests for dementia include the following.

The Stanford Proxy Test for Delirium (S-PTD)

The Stanford Proxy Test for Delirium (S-PTD)[11] is a screening tool for the exclusive use by nursing staff in both critical and non-critical patient populations which has excellent validity in detecting delirium.

Confusion Assessment Method (CAM)

This is the most widely used assessment tool in the field, and has been found to be both a sensitive and specific tool for delirium detection.

Single Question in Delirium (SQiD)

The simplicity of this test is appealing. Possible questions include:

- 'Do you think (name) has been more confused lately?'

- 'Have there been sudden changes in his behaviour?'

- 'Has he become more agitated?'

- 'Has he become more withdrawn?'

Asking the SQiD question on a regular basis can identify changes in a patient's condition, which could potentially be delirium. Family carers arguably know the older person best and can relate to patients in a way that health professionals might not be able to. Family carers will often notice subtle changes in the older person's cognition and behaviour. Recognising that a person is more confused than before should trigger escalation to medical staff and initiation of 4AT rapid assessment test for delirium.

4AT test

The 4As in 4AT stand for Arousal, Attention, Abbreviated Mental Test 4 and Acute change. It is shown in Figure 1.2.

The 4AT is a screening instrument designed for rapid initial assessment of delirium and cognitive impairment. The 4AT tool should be used for identifying patients with probable delirium in emergency department and acute hospital settings.

4AT

**Assessment test
for delirium &
cognitive impairment**

Patient name:
Date of birth:
Patient number:

Date: Time:

Tester:

[1] ALERTNESS		CIRCLE

This includes patients who may be markedly drowsy (e.g. difficult to rouse and/or obviously sleepy during assessment) or agitated/hyperactive. Observe the patient. If asleep, attempt to wake with speech or gentle touch on the shoulder. Ask the patient to state their name and address to assist rating.

Normal (fully alert, but not agitated, throughout assessment)	0
Mild sleepiness for <10 seconds after waking, then normal	0
Clearly abnormal	4

[2] AMT4
Age, date of birth, place (name of the hospital or building), current year

No mistakes	0
1 mistake	1
2 or more mistakes/untestable	2

[3] ATTENTION
Ask the patient: 'Please tell me the months of the year in backwards order, starting at December.' To assist initial understanding one prompt of 'What is the month before December?' is permitted.

Months of the year backwards		
	Achieves 7 months or more correctly	0
	Starts but scores <7 months/refuses to start	1
	Untestable (cannot start because unwell, drowsy, inattentive)	2

[4] ACUTE CHANGE OR FLUCTUATING COURSE
Evidence of significant change or fluctuation in: alertness, cognition, other mental function (e.g. paranoia, hallucinations) arising over the last 2 weeks and still evident in 24hrs)

No	0
Yes	4

4 or above: possible delirium +/– cognitive impairment
1–3: possible cognitive impairment
0: delirium or severe cognitive impairment unlikely (but delirium still possible if [4] information incomplete)

4AT SCORE [   ]

Figure 1.2 The 4AT[12]

SCORING

A score of 4 or more suggests delirium but is not diagnostic: more detailed assessment of mental status may be required to reach a diagnosis. A score of 1–3 suggests cognitive impairment and more detailed cognitive testing and informant history taking are required.

A score of 0 does not definitively exclude delirium or cognitive impairment: more detailed testing may be required depending on the clinical context. Items 1–3 are rated solely on observation of the patient at the time of assessment.

Item 4 requires information from one or more source(s) – for example, your own knowledge of the patient, other staff who know the patient, GP letter, case notes, carers. The tester should take account of communication difficulties – such as sensory impairment, dysphasia, lack of common language – when carrying out the test and interpreting the score.

Important properties include:

- It tests alertness, attention, AMT4 and acute history, and has a high sensitivity and specificity.

- It is brief and simple, and is freely available (see www.the4at.com).

- It is quick to complete, taking about two minutes.

- It results in accurate detection of delirium, defined according to standardised clinical criteria, and does not require specific clinical experience or preliminary training of assessors.

- It can be used with patients who are severely agitated.

- It is recommended in several pathways and guidelines and is in wide routine clinical use in the UK and internationally.

The 4AT has to date been evaluated in many validation studies with varying designs, reference standards, clinical populations and inclusion criteria; sensitivities are reported as 83–100% and specificities ranging from 70 to 99%.[13]

A recent NIHR report noted the following:[14]

A normal 4AT score reliably ruled out delirium. An abnormal score was also reasonably effective in detecting delirium, but staff still needed to follow up such patients with a full assessment. People with higher 4AT scores stayed in hospital longer and were more likely to die, and their treatment was more expensive.

Awareness of delirium

The overall knowledge of delirium can be low even in junior doctors. The publication of the **2019 SIGN guideline for delirium**[15] may have provided a stimulus for greater understanding of delirium among trainees, giving a clear national reference for the identification, investigation and management of patients with delirium. Implementing clinical guidelines requires all health professionals to change their personal and team practices to incorporate new actions into their practices.

Simulation-based learning, as reported by some, can provide the opportunity of practised experience in a controlled, reproducible fashion which can then be reflected upon at leisure. This is discussed further in Chapter 13.

A further significant policy shift initiative which may lead to an improvement in the recognition of delirium is the implementation of the dementia CQUIN (Commissioning for Quality and Innovation) target. This requires admitting staff to perform a cognitive assessment on all patients admitted as an emergency who are over the age of 75 with an aim to increase identification of patients with delirium and dementia.

The improvement of awareness of delirium has been greatly helped by the international societies EDA and ADS.

The **European Delirium Association** (EDA; www.europeandelirium association.com) was established in 2006 with the main aims of promoting knowledge of delirium, improving clinical management and providing support for research within Europe.

The **American Delirium Society** (ADS; www.americandeliriumsociety. org) was recently created with similar goals, underlining the importance of coordinating clinical and research efforts to reduce the impact of delirium on short- and long-term health outcomes.

The **Hospital Elder Life Program** (HELP; www.hospitalelderlifeprogram. org) is a comprehensive, evidence-based, patient-care programme that provides optimal care for older people in hospital.

The **Network for Investigation of Delirium: Unifying Scientists** (NIDUS; www.deliriumnetwork.org) was created to provide education and resources about delirium and to support a collaborative network to advance scientific research on the causes, mechanisms, outcomes, diagnosis, prevention and treatment of delirium in older adults.

Another excellent source of information is **MindEd for Families** (www. mindedforfamilies.org.uk). This website includes videos and information to raise awareness of what delirium is and to help older people and those around them learn how to deal with it.

See also **Royal College of Psychiatrists** (www.rcpsych.ac.uk/mental-health/problems-disorders/delirium), which provides information on signs and symptoms, treatment and what may happen after a person has had delirium.

What is it actually like to have delirium?

Box 1.1 shows some possibilities. Once you've met one person with delirium, you've only met one person with delirium.

BOX 1.1 WHAT DOES IT FEEL LIKE TO BE EXPERIENCING DELIRIUM?

- Find it difficult to concentrate on conversations or be slow to answer
- Feel muddled and mistake where you are
- Experience seeing or hearing things which nobody else can or mistake real objects for something else
- Be more restless, agitated and over-active or more often excessively sleepy
- Be reluctant to eat and drink
- Be awake more during the night
- Be sleepy and slow to respond
- Have frightening dreams
- Struggle to understand and cooperate with what people are asking you to do
- See people or things that aren't there
- Hear voices or noises which aren't actually present
- Experience rather rapid mood swings
- Be less aware of what is going on around you
- Be unsure about where you are or what you are doing there
- Worry that other people are trying to harm you
- Have a temporary change in personality and behaviour, including being very agitated or restless, unable to sit still and wandering about
- Be very slow or sleepy sleep during the day but wake up at night
- Be more confused at some times than at others

Fluctuation of delirium

ICD-10 defines delirium as:[16]

> An etiologically nonspecific organic cerebral syndrome characterised by concurrent disturbances of consciousness and attention, perception, thinking, memory, psychomotor behaviour, emotion, and the sleep–wake schedule. The duration is variable and the degree of severity ranges from mild to very severe.

Fluctuation is a defining characteristic of delirium, and chart-based methods may capture delirium that was not present during the time when clerking took place but that developed at a different time of day (e.g. during the night shift).

The fluctuating nature of delirium means that serial assessment is required. One difficulty is that repetition of cognitive assessments will be affected by a practice effect.

A 'chart-review method' that does not require direct patient interaction and that covers the 24-hour period and has been validated requires hand-searches of all relevant records (e.g. nursing and physician notes) and relies on clinical judgement.

We do not know, as yet, the neural mechanism of this fluctuation, although some scholarly articles, such as that of Matar and colleagues, have recently made some useful inroads.[17] This fluctuation of cognitive, behavioural or physical symptoms poses practical problems for assessment of patient safety.

Definition

Working definitions of delirium vary, although diagnostic criteria evolve.

Broadly speaking, delirium is an acute decline in mental functioning with confusion, overactivity or underactivity, and distress. It can be precipitated by acute medical illness, by surgery or by medicines or medication withdrawal. Most patients recover in a few days to a few weeks. Delirium is not the same as dementia, which is chronic and generally irreversible. The manifestations of delirium can be cognitive, emotional, motor, affective or motivational. It can arise as a physiological consequence of a medical condition, substance withdrawal or some other form of toxic state.

Characterising delirium

It is argued that the **fundamental phenomenology of delirium** is as follows:[18]

- cognitive deficits

- attentional deficits

- circadian rhythm dysregulation and fragmentation of the sleep–wake cycle

- emotional dysregulation *and*

- psychomotor dysregulation.

In 2000, Mesulam[19] proposed that two brain networks may be disrupted in patients with delirium. These networks include 'bottom-up', afferent projections of the ascending reticular activating system, a system involved in wakefulness and arousal; and 'top-down' modulation of attention by frontal, parietal and limbic cortices.

The patient with delirium may not able to respond to or recognise the environment appropriately. The abrupt disorientation in time and space, in association with an inability to recall references, either spontaneously or after suggestion, prevents the subject from processing sensibly the context of perceptual information. Eventually, this altered perception may cause an increased level of anxiety and agitation.

Delirium may be associated with alterations of the sleep–wake cycle, featured in daytime sleeping and sleepless nights. There is a close relationship between the disruption of the circadian system and the development of delirium. This might ultimately suggest a strong association between melatonin daily rhythms and delirium onset, thus suggesting that melatonin daily rhythm may be a useful predictive strategy for developing delirium, or may simply suggest an overall malfunction of the hypothalamus.

A quick look for a possible cause

A mnemonic that nurses can use when looking after patients with signs of delirium is **PINCH ME.**

It prompts consideration of the root causes of delirium, which is helpful as identifying these can lead to quicker interventions and treatment.

PINCH ME forms part of the nursing dementia and delirium bundles in some Trusts currently.[20]

Pain
Infection
Nutrition
Constipation
Hydration/hypoxia
Medication
Environment

Common types of delirium

It is helpful to classify delirium according to predominant symptoms, likely aetiology and context of presentation. Like dementia, acknowledging these specific sub-classifications of delirium provides much more precision to the discussion and anticipation of symptoms:

- hyperactive delirium

- hypoactive delirium

- mixed delirium

- subsyndromal delirium

- delirium superimposed on dementia

- emergence delirium

- excited delirium

- persistent delirium

- paediatric delirium.

The features of delirium sometimes cluster, allowing for subtyping – for example, into hyperactive, hypoactive and mixed categories, or subtypes where cognitive disturbance or altered higher-order thinking, or altered circadian functions predominate. Future clarity on the epidemiology of the common subtypes will prove to be helpful.

These putative clinical variants share core cognitive impairment but may differ in terms of underlying aetiology and outcomes, with hypoactive presentations linked to poorer prognosis.

In patients who are considered to be experiencing delirium, an important yet unresolved issue is whether they all suffer from the same condition. There still remains the possibility of a 'final common pathway'.[21] The substrate of this hypothetical pathway is unclear, and there is a lack of comparison studies on clinical features in delirium due to different aetiologies and different settings. Studies on different delirium aetiologies are difficult to perform as it is usually impossible to assign one specific cause for delirium.

People can appear to 'change' so quickly with delirium. That's why it's so scary. We do not know whether the hyperactive, hypoactive and mixed subtypes of delirium are all part of essentially the same phenotype. We do not even know how or if the subtypes alternate during one episode of delirium.

The recognised 'subtypes' of delirium are described below:

1. **Hyperactive subtype:** Increased psychomotor activity and an exaggerated response to external stimuli are prominent features of hyperactive delirium. A person with hyperactive delirium may experience vivid hallucinations and illusions, paranoia and aggressive behaviour. People with a hyperactive form of delirium can experience symptoms which lead them to feel fearful of or threatened by those

caring for them. They may actively resist care, become agitated or even try to abscond.

2. **Hypoactive subtype:** On the other hand, it is harder to recognise hypoactive delirium because it presents as reduced psychomotor activity, decreased alertness and excessive somnolence. Hypoactive delirium, seemingly less of a management problem, nevertheless hampers cooperation with nursing, physical care and other activities.

   Hypoactive delirium can look a lot like severe depression – a patient might suddenly look very tearful, express uncertainty about the future and burst into tears. Closer questioning will, however, reveal signs of inattention and decreased awareness of the environment. People with hypoactive delirium who are sleepy and lethargic may forget to drink, be unable to feed themselves and can easily become dehydrated.

   Hypoactive delirium, due to lack of interest in food, drink or moving, can also look a lot like end of life.

3. The **mixed subtype** presents with symptoms of both hyperactive and hypoactive delirium. Limited awareness about the syndrome and especially how this can vary in presentation may be one reason that delirium is under-recognised, misdiagnosed and under-reported in practice.

The hypoactive, hyperactive and mixed subtypes of delirium differently impact patient management and prognosis, yet detailed projections of their timelines are as yet not forthcoming; in a recent large observational cohort study, the mixed subtype predicted more severe and persistent delirium, and the hypoactive subtype appeared to be perhaps less responsive to management than the hyperactive subtype.[22]

Subsyndromal delirium

Subsyndromal delirium (SSD) is characterised by a milder state of delirium, including one or more symptoms of delirium, without the features of the full syndrome. SSD has been a more controversial clinical entity to discuss than full syndrome delirium. Although SSD arguably does not have universally agreed and clearly defined descriptive diagnostic criteria, it is listed in the neurocognitive disorder section of DSM-5 as 'attenuated delirium syndrome'.[23] Whether SSD may progress to delirium and whether early intervention will prevent the development of delirium remain unknown.

Both delirium and SSD in the intensive care unit (ICU) are recognised as determinants for long-term functional disability and cognitive impairment, although relatively few studies on SSD outcomes have been reported.[24] A high incidence of SSD is observed in critically ill patients. Patient with SSD must be promptly identified and treated due to the risk of progression to delirium.

Further studies and consensus are needed to define better SSD.

Delirium superimposed on dementia

DSM-5 states that delirium should not be diagnosed when symptoms can be 'better accounted for by a pre-existing, established, or evolving dementia'.[25] This leads to the notion that 'delirium superimposed on dementia' (DSD) is a delirium occurring in a patient already with a dementia process. However, this simple notion leads to interpretational difficulties for both practitioners and researchers. When compared with delirium alone, DSD is associated with worse outcomes, including increased walking dependence, institutionalisation and mortality, along with worsening of existing cognitive decline. The lack of standardisation in the assessment of DSD may have potential significant clinical and research implications.

Delirium prolongs hospitalisation for patients with dementia.[26] Thus, interventions to increase early detection of delirium have the potential to decrease the severity and duration of delirium and to prevent unnecessary suffering and costs from complications and unnecessary readmissions to the hospital.

There is considerable uncertainty regarding the assessment of DSD and, partly as a consequence of this, it is sometimes missed. People who are older with dementia and who are institutionalised are at increased risk of developing delirium when hospitalised. Results of studies on DSD prevalence assessment are extremely variable; frequently, delirium symptoms are erroneously attributed to the underlying dementia.

A word of caution, however. Delirium and dementia of Lewy bodies (DLB) share a number of clinical similarities, including global impairment of cognition, fluctuations in attention and perceptual abnormalities. Delirium is a frequent presenting feature of DLB.[27]

Delirium is perhaps the most common fluctuating encephalopathy encountered in general medical practice, and many of its cardinal features mirror the fluctuating phenotype of DLB.[28]

The identification of delirium in DLB patients is particularly challenging, although recurrent delirium is much more common prior to the onset of dementia in DLB than in Alzheimer's disease. It has been noted that DLB can first present as cognitive impairment, delirium or a psychiatric problem such as psychosis or depression.[29]

Emergence delirium

Emergence from anaesthesia is a final stage of anaesthesia featuring the transition from unconsciousness to complete wakefulness and regaining of consciousness. From a neuroscientific perspective, it is hypothesised that the processes involved cannot be simply considered as reverse events which occur in the induction of anaesthesia.

Emergence delirium is a clinical condition in which patients are 'awake' but experience alterations in orientation and mental status that range from confusion and lethargy to violent, dangerous behaviour.

In older patients, this form of delirium may be prolonged and may not be diagnosed until even a day post-operatively. It takes longer for emergence delirium symptoms to occur, possibly because older adults metabolise anaesthesia medications at a slower rate. Although most patients experiencing emergence delirium display periods of excitement alternating with periods of lethargy, older adult patients may appear restless without notable changes in physical behaviour.

Excited delirium

Excited delirium is a wide-ranging phenotype involving agitation, aggression and paranoia, intolerance to pain, unexpected physical strength, failure to fatigue despite constant physical activity, lack of clothing, tachypnoea, profuse sweating, elevated temperature, and failure to respond appropriately to external presences, including the police. These cases of excited delirium can often involve men in their 30s after cocaine, methamphetamine or ecstasy abuse.

Cases of extreme agitation have been described since the 19th century, with Luther Bell's eponymous 'Bell's mania' being described in October 1849.[30] The term 'excited delirium' syndrome was coined in the 1980s, after a spate of deaths of individuals in custody or during arrests following extreme agitation.[31]

The difficulty surrounding the clinical identification of excited delirium is that the spectrum of behaviours and signs overlap with so many other clinical disease processes.

This subject is explored further in Chapter 2.

Persistent delirium

In **persistent delirium**, delirium can persist for three months or more in around one in five cases.

Whenever it happens, it tends to be rather ominous. A previous study found that patients whose delirium persisted were nearly three times more likely to die during the one-year follow-up compared with patients who resolved their delirium, even after adjusting for the compounding effects of age, gender, comorbidity, functional status and dementia.[32]

Patients with persistent delirium are at especially high risk of misdiagnosis and mismanagement: they are often labelled as having 'confusion' and not given a formal diagnosis. This can lead to a lack of thoroughness in searching for unaddressed causes, and to unsuccessful efforts to rehabilitate and provide an appropriate environment. Ultimately, many patients with persistent delirium are inappropriately put into residential care, with the diagnosis only apparent if the patient recovers.

The poor prognosis of delirium among older hospital patients may be because many of these patients do not recover from delirium; the persistence of delirium, rather than the occurrence of an episode of delirium *per se*, accounts for many of the adverse outcomes.[33]

Paediatric delirium

Paediatric delirium had long been considered a common but relatively inconsequential neuropsychiatric concomitant of physical illness, but in recent years this notion has been challenged. Despite childhood delirium remaining a severely neglected area of research, an emerging literature is beginning to outline both continuities and discontinuities with the adult syndrome.

It is argued that there exist symptoms and signs of delirium that are similar across the age span, although certain features such as irritability are reported more commonly in children, while other features such as delusions are reported less commonly.

Delirium in children is an often under-recognised but serious complication of hospitalisation.

Developmental regression has also been suggested as a relatively unique feature of delirium in children and adolescents. Long-term cognitive dysfunction and schooling are therefore of concern.

Risk factors for developing paediatric delirium have been well characterised and include younger age, male gender, acute neurological injury, pre-existing cognitive impairment or developmental delay at baseline, and pre-existing emotional and behavioural problems.[34] Exacerbating environmental factors include physical restraints, high noise levels, poor lighting and frequent staff changes.

Paediatric delirium may be an indicator of worsening clinical status in children and is associated with high mortality and morbidity in children of all ages and with post-traumatic stress disorder. Its identification is therefore essential.

Paediatric delirium in the ICU has been associated with longer length of stay.[35]

Delirium is an important and significant medical emergency

Delirium is among the most common of medical emergencies.

Appropriately recognising and diagnosing delirium upon onset is crucial because the condition is reversible and linked to possibly life-threatening disorders. Delirium should be considered an emergency medical condition that requires an appraisal of the clinical care up until that point, as well as an indicator that a more intensive clinical approach might be needed. When the possibility of delirium is considered early, physicians tend to protect the patient from this risk, being forced to rule out organic causes of symptoms before starting any pharmacological treatment.

Delirium is commonly overlooked or misattributed to dementia, depression or simply old age (i.e. older patients are expected to get confused in the hospital).

There might be several reasons for this lack of recognition.

Delirium as a potential medical emergency has been under-appreciated. Many physicians are not aware that, in elderly patients, delirium may be the *sole manifestation* of life-threatening illness, such as stroke, sepsis or myocardial infarction. Also, delirium is not often regarded as an important clinical syndrome because its varied and multiple aetiologies in the elderly might be 'atypical' of the classical disease presentation. The fluctuating nature of delirium may confound the diagnosis, since clinicians may spot lucid intervals which are characteristic of the syndrome.

There is some cause for optimism with improvements in many aspects of the understanding of delirium, possibly as a consequence of major national and international initiatives. However, the core diagnostic criteria for delirium remain poorly understood and may require further epidemiological analysis.

Early detection of delirium is important

The most important step in delirium management is **early recognition**. The reason for this is that if delirium is not diagnosed promptly, it is unlikely that any effort will be made to reverse it or mitigate its effects. Once delirium is suspected, the first urgent aim is to identify the underlying aetiology. Often this can be achieved by a systematic assessment of the presence of known risk factors.

Delirium is both common and dangerous, but current evidence suggests it is also preventable in about one-third of cases, hence the growing emphasis on the adoption of multicomponent delirium prevention interventions. Raising awareness and training of nurses can prevent a substantial proportion of delirium cases. Research shows that educational initiatives have a helping role in detection of delirium (Chapter 13).

Minimisation and/or elimination of predisposing and precipitating factors is the natural main strategy in treating and preventing delirium. Management should focus on improving the patient's health status and reducing the risk of adverse outcomes.

Delirium has poor outcomes if missed

Knowledge and understanding of the significance of delirium, including its impact on patient distress and outcomes, are critical to the engagement of staff in delirium detection. It is recognised that delirium at any stage of the acute illness of hospital inpatients is associated with a range of adverse outcomes, even after statistically adjusting for predisposing factors such as disability and cognitive impairment and severity of illness. Detection of delirium is important because of the associated morbidity and mortality: although most patients with delirium recover, some progress to stupor, coma, seizures or death. Patients may die because of failure to treat the associated medical condition or from the delirium itself (although the mechanism is currently unclear).

A core pathology?

Delirium is a complex neuroscientific syndrome caused by the transient disruption of normal neuronal activity secondary to systemic disturbances. Given the multifactorial aetiology of delirium, each individual episode of delirium is likely to have a unique set of component contributors; however, how the contributing factors all interact remains an enigma.

The most comprehensive update on all literature and research on the pathophysiology of delirium was written by Trepacz and Van der Mast in 2002. The authors pose that certain neuroanatomical and neurotransmitter systems may represent a 'final common neural pathway' for the diverse aetiologies of delirium.[36] The kernel of this view stems from the notion that despite such a diversity of predisposing and triggering factors, there is a striking similarity in the manifestation of the clinical symptoms of the delirium syndromes.

Genetics of delirium

Since delirium is a multifactorial disorder, the genetic make-up alone is likely insufficient to identify high-risk patients. Individual differences, including genetic factors and level of cognitive reserve, might contribute to the severity of delirium in older adults with dementia.[37]

Candidate **genome-wide association studies** (GWAS) are relatively quick and relatively inexpensive to perform. They can test the effect of genetic variants of a potential contributing gene (the candidate gene) in unrelated cases and controls. Interleukin receptors may be implicated in GWAS, and this seems a sensible place to start as the inflammatory response might be involved in delirium.[38] The field of genetics has already acquired a prominent place in pathophysiological research in neuropsychiatric disorders.[39] Genetic research offers new possibilities in elucidating the underlying neural substrates of delirium.

Epigenetics refers to heritable changes in phenotype or gene expression caused by mechanisms other than changes in the underlying DNA sequence. Biological, chemical and physical factors as well as personal factors, such as cultural and educational backgrounds, can influence gene functioning. Environmental factors, such as stress, play a major role in psychiatric disorders by inducing stable changes in gene expression; potentially, therefore, there is a biologically plausible mechanism.

The relationship between delirium and stress

Delirium might constitute an example of an 'aberrant stress response', comprising a group of responses that are somehow abnormal in certain individuals, such that responses that are typically adaptive under normal circumstances become maladaptive. In this framing, 'stress' broadly refers to the sympathetic nervous system, hypothalamic–pituitary–adrenal axis, inflammatory pathways and other systems activated in response to an acute threat or 'stressor'. The term 'aberrant' is used because the stress response may be exaggerated and manifestly has adverse effects on the brain.

The hormone **cortisol** is an associated risk factor of brain dysfunction in patients with severe sepsis and septic shock. Cortisol has even been suggested to be a 'biomarker' for the diagnosis of delirium.[40] It has been reported that excessive cortisol or catecholamine release is involved in the development of delirium in severe sepsis, Cushing's disease and psychosis.[41] Levels of cortisol in the cerebrospinal fluid more closely reflect brain exposure to cortisol. The psychophysiological stress associated with hospitalisation may also lead to sustained effects following hospital discharge, resulting in impaired short-term recovery and increased long-term healthcare utilisation.[42]

The 'systems integration failure hypothesis'

Our historic lack of understanding of the pathophysiological changes of delirium potentially limits our ability to develop new treatments and prevention strategies.

On the basis of an extensive literature search, a newly proposed theory, the systems integration failure hypothesis, was developed by José R. Maldonado to bring together the most salient previously described theories, by combining the various contributions from each into a complex web of pathway. The 'systems integration failure hypothesis' elegantly proposes that the specific combination of cognitive and behavioural manifestations of the specific delirium picture result from a combination of neurotransmitter dysfunction, variability in integration and processing of sensorimotor information, and the degree of breakdown in neuronal network connectivity.[43]

Delirium occurs in a number of diverse care settings

Is delirium in the nursing home fundamentally the same entity as delirium in the ICU?

Delirium occurs in all care settings.

Improving clinical practice involves teamwork from individuals to whole systems.

The incidence and prevalence of delirium depends on both the age group and clinical setting. The prevalence of delirium is highest in older hospitalised individuals and 'varies depending on the patient characteristics, setting of care, and sensitivity of the detection method'.[44] Delirium can occur in any of the possible care settings where delirium might occur – for example, in a person's own home, a hospice or a care home. It is thought to happen to around 15% of adult acute general patients, 30% of acute geriatrics patients, 50% of ICU patients and 50% patients following hip fracture surgery.[45]

Care-home residents have a high prevalence of dementia and therefore may be at high risk of delirium. Care staff are well placed to detect changes in behaviour or arousal due to their close contact with residents, but may not be trained to recognise this as delirium and take the appropriate action. Early detection and management may prevent inappropriate out-of-hours GP contact or hospital admission.

Prevalence of delirium is higher in particular groups, such as older patients and patients in the ICU.

ICU delirium is defined as 'an altered state of consciousness featuring disordered attention, impaired cognition, altered psychomotor activity (increased or decreased) and disorder of the sleep–wake cycle'.[46]

It has an acute onset and is thought to be reversible, although long-term cognitive impairment is common after diagnosis of ICU delirium. ICU delirium can be very distressing for both the patients themselves and any carers who happen to be supporting them. Elderly patients with hip fractures are particularly vulnerable to developing post-operative delirium, with an incidence ranging between 5% and 61%.[47] Hip fractures also signify a pre-morbid decrease in function. A subsequent episode of perioperative delirium may result in a lifelong functional impairment and increased mortality.

As the underlying mechanism of delirium is likely to be heterogeneous, it is not surprising that the epidemiology and associated risk factors vary from one setting to another. Importantly, the predisposing and precipitating factors that place a patient at high risk in one setting maybe non-existent in others.

Hospitalisation

Hospitalisation may lead to complications that are not specific to the presenting illness, often called geriatric syndromes – conditions with a higher prevalence in older than younger people, multifactorial aetiology, shared risk factors and negative effects on outcomes. Delirium has become officially noted for that very reason; it is now recognised by the Australian Commission for Safety and Quality in Health Care as a hospital-acquired complication of hospitalisation.[48] Acute hospital inpatient populations are becoming older and this presents the potential for poorer health outcomes. Factors such as a rising prevalence of chronic health conditions, increasing use of polypharmacy and cognitive and functional decline are associated with increased risk of 'healthcare-related harm'.[49]

It is abundantly clear that patients hospitalised for medical illnesses and surgical procedures are at risk of delirium. Up to one in three people admitted to hospital experience delirium at some time during their stay. Delirium may occur at any time during a hospital stay, so clinicians should have a fairly low threshold for spotting it during the course of the patient's illness. Indeed, with earlier hospital discharges, it is likely that post-discharge delirium (at home or in the nursing home) may be more common than is generally realised.

History and examination

A thorough history is required to elicit possible delirium precipitants, which themselves can be numerous and varied in one individual.

'THINK DELIRIUM' MEMORY AID

Drugs/**D**ehydration

Electrolyte imbalance

Level of pain

Infection/Inflammation

Respiratory failure

Impaction of faeces

Urine retention

Metabolic disorder/**M**yocardial infarction

Attention should be paid to preventing modifiable factors and attenuating the impact of non-modifiable risk factors. Patients with delirium often struggle to follow the actual instructions of a traditional neurological exam, yet careful observation at the bedside may identify signs attributable to the underlying aetiology.

A full assessment of all prescriptions, including very recent changes, over-the-counter or homeopathic remedies, and adherence/compliance is required.

Many medicines have deliriogenic side effects, particularly those with anti-cholinergic profiles. Sudden withdrawal of opiates, benzodiazepines and other sedatives may also cause delirium; if these medications are to be stopped, specialist knowledge is advisable. Over-reliance on investigation in place of a thorough collateral history and careful examination can cause diagnostic delay, and the transfer across the hospital for multiple tests can cause added harm.

Constipation, urinary retention and medications are common causes of delirium that may not cause abnormality in blood tests.

> **ADVICE GIVEN TO PATIENTS**
> Try to avoid constipation by eating plenty of fruit and vegetables and staying as mobile as you can. You can ask for laxatives.

Investigations should be pragmatic, with the routine use of simple tests. A stepwise approach to further investigation is best directed by the clinical history and examination findings.

The actual development of delirium

The development of delirium involves the complex inter-relationship between a vulnerable patient with multiple predisposing factors and exposure to precipitating factors. Predisposing factors vary and will amass with time. Research in the fields of ageing and dementia urge a need to understand the importance of complexity in deficit accumulation during the life course.[50]

Currently, there is very little published evidence on the natural history – or, indeed, time course – of variants of delirium. One day, it may be necessary to link this to physiological, biochemical or functional changes, *inter alia*.

Risk factors for delirium can be classified into two groups: baseline factors that *predispose* patients to delirium and acute factors that *precipitate* delirium. There is a belief that, with a higher number of predisposing factors, fewer precipitating factors are needed for delirium to develop. The underlying aetiology can be classified according to the presence of predisposing and triggering factors. The predisposing factors characterise those individuals that are more likely to develop delirium, while the presence of triggering factors subsequently establishes the disorder.

But no one actually knows what 'flicks' the neural mechanism into a type of delirium once that sufficient threshold of precipitating and predisposing factors has been met in any one individual. It could be possible, for example, that one patient will always experience delirium after surgery but never after infection.

In a recently published prospective cohort study of 1487 neurological patients,[51] the most relevant predisposing factor was substance-use disorders, followed by age over 65 years and pre-existing dementias or degenerative disorders. Meningitis was the most relevant precipitating factor with a more than 20-times increased risk for delirium, followed by acute renal failure increasing the odds tenfold, whereas intracranial haemorrhage and sepsis-related disorders also increased the risk of delirium.

Predisposing factors

Examples of some typical **predisposing factors** are shown in Box 1.2.

BOX 1.2 PREDISPOSING FACTORS

- Chronic hepatic or renal impairment
- Cognitive impairment and dementia
- Current or past alcohol abuse
- Demyelinating conditions
- Depression
- Diabetes mellitus
- Dysphagia
- Epilepsy
- Frailty
- Functional dependency
- Hearing impairment
- History of delirium
- History of stroke or other neurological disorder
- Hydrocephalus
- Inadequate hydration
- Male sex
- Malnutrition
- Multiple comorbidities
- Old and very old age (>90 years)
- Polypharmacy
- Pre-existing cognitive deficit or dementia
- Previous episode of delirium
- Stroke
- Visual impairment

Patients should be advised to avoid illness through smoking cessation, a balanced diet, regular exercise, adequate hydration and vaccinations to prevent influenza and pneumonia. Caution should be exercised with medication, especially sleep aids, and physicians should review medicines periodically.

ADVICE GIVEN TO PATIENTS

- If you smoke, talk to a doctor or nurse about nicotine patches while you're in hospital as nicotine withdrawal can contribute to delirium.
- If you drink several alcoholic drinks most days, discuss this with a doctor or nurse as alcohol withdrawal can cause delirium.

Delirium is more common in those with a pre-existing organic brain syndrome or dementia, and may co-exist with disorders such as depression that are also common in older people. Patients with dementia are five times more likely to develop delirium. Chronic medical illnesses, comorbidity, disease severity and functional impairment also serve as predisposing factors to delirium. Thyroid or adrenal dysfunction, alcohol dependence, diabetes mellitus, burns, cancer, malnutrition with reduced plasma binding, vitamin B_1 deficiency, vitamin B_{12} deficiency and pellagra may also contribute to the development of delirium.

Environmental factors that lead to altered sensory perceptions, including sensory impairment – for example, inadequate lighting, increased noise levels, blindness or poor hearing, sleep deprivation, stress or major environmental factors – all contribute to the development of delirium or the worsening of delirium.

It is worth noting that certain factors imposed by the care environment, such as immobility including physical restraint use and the use of indwelling bladder catheters, may greatly increase the risk of delirium and functional decline.

Triggering or precipitating factors

The syndrome of delirium is better thought of as having a multifactorial aetiology, as is often the case in most medically ill patients.

Examples of some typical **triggering or precipitating factors** is shown in Box 1.3.

BOX 1.3 TRIGGERING OR PRECIPITATING FACTORS

- Anaemia
- Autoimmune diseases including paraneoplastic phenomena
- Cardiological conditions
- Constipation
- Decreased amount of sleep

- Dehydration and malnutrition
- Drugs – including acute withdrawal, introduction of a new medication and polypharmacy
- Electrolyte imbalance
- Endocrine and metabolic conditions
- Falls
- Hospital admission
- Hypoglycaemia
- Infection
- Major surgical operation
- Neurological conditions
- Pain
- Pressure ulcers
- Respiratory conditions
- Suddenly stopping drugs and/or alcohol
- Unfamiliar environment
- Unmanaged epilepsy
- Urinary catheter

Most older patients may have several triggering factors, and although only one triggering event is usually located, it is more common for several co-existing factors to be implicated.

A major part of treating people with delirium is treating the underlying precipitants or causes. A structured approach should be taken to identify, where possible, the issues contributing to delirium for an individual. These include a comprehensive assessment, which might also include a good history from the person, a collateral or informant history, and full clinical examination.

People with dementia experiencing pain at rest may be more likely to be delirious and can experience pain for a substantial part of their stay in hospital without being able to communicate this pain. Delirium and pain are both potentially identifiable and manageable, but both are associated with numerous adverse outcomes, including increased length of stay in hospital, mortality and institutionalisation. It can be difficult to ascertain the extent to which a patient is impaired, especially if he is cognitively impaired and has communication difficulties.

Both room transfers and a long time spent in the emergency department can be stressful events that might induce aberrant stress responses eventually contributing to delirium. Due to the substantial impact of delirium and the increasing number of older patients at risk for delirium in strained and crowded hospitals, there is a need to further explore the associations between potentially stressful environmental factors in the hospital care pathway itself and delirium.

Clinically, suspicion of an infectious process must remain high, especially in older patients who may not be able to mount the appropriate immunological response. Infections are a much more frequent precipitating factor for delirium in community-dwelling patients than in in-hospital patients.[52]

Cardiovascular events such as acute myocardial infarction, congestive heart failure, cardiac arrest and cardiogenic shock commonly present with delirium. Low perfusion states, hypoxia, metabolic disorders such as dehydration, hypo- or hyperglycaemia, hyper- or hypo-natraemia, hypercalcaemia and toxic confusional states such as alcohol or drug intoxication or withdrawal states can also contribute to the development of delirium.

Patients who have experienced a stroke are particularly vulnerable to delirium as a consequence of the direct cerebral insult and the occurrence of one or more acknowledged risk factors, such as cognitive, visual and functional impairments. Delirium episodes in this population have been documented as negatively affecting outcomes both in the short and in the long term. Ischaemic injury to white matter tracts is increasingly recognised as playing a key role in age-related cognitive decline and dementias, and certain molecular mechanisms might be at play.[53]

Infections as triggering or precipitating factors

Two engrained ageist 'attitudes':
- Confused old people must have a urinary tract infection (UTI).
- Old people are expected to get confused.

Infectious diseases account for widespread morbidity and mortality among the elderly; for example, in 2012 alone, infectious diseases accounted for 3.1 million visits made by elders to U.S. emergency departments.[54] Accurate infection diagnosis is complicated by the absence of typical symptoms found in younger adults, lack of accurate diagnostic criteria, absence of timely culture results, long-term micro-organism colonisation and comorbidities.

Both over-diagnosis and under-diagnosis of a potential infective 'cause' of delirium can occur. Over-diagnosis may result in increased costs, inappropriate antibiotic use, missed alternative diagnoses and avoidable admissions. Under-diagnosis can result in failure to adequately treat bacterial infections. Despite new onset or worsening of confusion being a non-specific symptom, it continues to be the most common reason for suspecting a lower UTI in elderly patients, often leading to antibiotic treatment.

The diagnosis of UTI is further complicated by the high prevalence of asymptomatic bacteriuria, particularly in nursing-home residents,. Treatment of asymptomatic bacteriuria and candiduria remains a leading reason for unnecessary antimicrobial use among hospitalised patients.[55]

Few studies have directly examined the association between UTI and delirium. Since no randomised controlled trials have evaluated this association, it is difficult to elucidate how and why UTIs can cause delirium and how successful treatment of UTI can lead to improvement in symptoms of delirium.[56] Delirium may be common in care homes due to the high prevalence of dementia – a key delirium risk factor.[57] Care-home staff are particularly well placed to detect changes in residents' behaviour that may indicate onset of delirium. However, many diagnostic tools for detection of delirium require time and expertise to administer and this limits their utility for use in routine care.

Predisposing cognitive impairment

The significance of the finding of a high proportion of people with delirium having prior undiagnosed cognitive impairment is that not only is delirium an important diagnosis to make in older patients admitted to hospital, but it also presents a strong opportunity to identify cognitive impairment.

A timely diagnosis of dementia during hospital admission may ameliorate adverse events associated with a hospital stay, allow suitable resource allocation, such as signposting to a cohort ward, or trigger a comprehensive geriatric assessment. In the longer term, diagnosing patients with long-term cognitive impairments allows identification of those who would benefit from appropriate risk prevention mechanisms. Individuals could then be counselled, advised and offered post-diagnostic support, or offered the opportunity to participate in research.

Detecting any sort of cognitive impairment is a prerequisite for high-quality clinical care because of the multiple immediate implications of cognitive impairment for patients and staff, including ensuring adequate communication with patients and their families, and doing careful assessment of capacity to provide valid consent for clinical procedures. It is also imperative to avoid giving treatments because of lack of valid consent.

The **IQCODE**[58] can be used to assess if a patient had a pre-existing cognitive impairment. The IQCODE is a widely used validated questionnaire, including in delirium studies, which allows estimation of whether or not an individual has a pre-existing cognitive impairment. It is administered to the nearest relative or carer and takes five minutes to complete.

The APOE4 polymorphism, which has an allele frequency of approximately 14%,[59] has been identified as a major susceptibility factor for late-onset Alzheimer's disease and is also independently associated with poor neurological outcome after closed-head injury and intracranial haemorrhage. How APOE4 polymorphism is relevant to delirium needs more explaining.

Taking into account the influence of pre-existing cognitive impairment is an important issue in genetic studies on delirium in the elderly.

Post-operative delirium and cognitive dysfunction

Prevention, early identification and treatment of post-operative complications are important.

Post-operative delirium is a serious and common complication of major surgery, especially for older patients.

The prevalence of post-operative delirium varies from 15% to 53% in older individuals, depending on the settings and populations; it is in any case too high to be neglected.[60] After an initial episode of delirium, post-episode treatment or intervention may have little effect on severity, duration or likelihood of recurrence.[61]

Some factors involved in the phenomenon of post-operative delirium are shown in Box 1.4.

BOX 1.4 POST-OPERATIVE DELIRIUM

- Individual patient factors preoperatively: age, preexisting cognitive deficit, frailty, previous episode of delirium.

- Evidence suggests that interventions that reduce sensory deficits, immobility, sleep disturbance, dehydration and cognitive impairment might perhaps reduce the number of episodes of delirium and their duration.

- Perioperative period factors – e.g. type of operation, duration of operation, physiological or metabolic disturbances, other intervening factors.

- Careful specialist advice needs to be taken regarding minimisation of exposure to drugs and to reduce doses or stop administration of high-risk compounds especially during high-risk periods, such as the perioperative period.

Wider significance

In addition to the high prevalence, the prognosis of delirium is very poor (this is considered more fully in Chapter 8).

Before its onset, delirium is assumed to be preventable in 30–40% of cases,[62] which emphasises the importance of attention for primary prevention and prevention of downstream distal outcomes. This can be achieved by interventions tackling risk factors, such as adequate pain management, hearing or visual aids, sleep enhancement, exercise training or dietary advice.

The use of a **'bundled approach'** to reduce delirium rates has also been successful. Bundles of care are a set of three to five independent, evidence-based interventions that, when implemented together, result in significantly better outcomes than when implemented individually. One study[63] has reported that surgical patients without pre-morbid dementia or functional decline benefited most from any intervention, whereas multicomponent interventions were most effective for patients who exhibited one or two risk factors of delirium, specifically visual impairment, severe illness and cognitive impairment. Failure to assess pre-operative cognitive impairment is hard to justify.

Identifying the presence of cognitive impairment in older adults presenting for elective surgery assists calculating the cost/benefit ratio of a procedure, and has repercussions for the meaning of informed consent for an intervention. Cognitive impairment is not a standard or routine part of pre-operative risk stratification of the surgical patient. Events experienced during surgery, including anaesthesia and trauma, can contribute to the development of a systemic inflammatory response that can cause multi-organ dysfunction. Post-surgical neuroinflammation is a documented phenomenon that results in changes in the structure and function of both nerves and synapses.

Prevention and risk reduction

According to the journal *Nature*:[64]

Disease prevention is a procedure through which individuals, particularly those with risk factors for a disease, are treated in order to prevent a disease from occurring. Treatment normally begins either before signs and symptoms of the disease occur, or shortly thereafter. Treatment can include patient education, lifestyle modification, and drugs.

Prevention therefore fundamentally involves reducing the risk of adverse outcomes, such as the loss of patient autonomy, development of comorbid illnesses and/or death as a result of disease.[65]

The original delirium prevention program, the Hospital Elder Life Program or HELP,[66] is a comprehensive patient-care programme that prevents delirium and ensures optimal care for older adults. An interdisciplinary team and highly trained volunteers use a multicomponent intervention strategy targeted to prevent delirium which includes protocols addressing:

- daily orientation and therapeutic activities to keep patients cognitively engaged

- early mobilisation to maintain physical activity

- feeding assistance and hydration

- hearing and vision adaptations

- non-pharmacological sleep assistance (relaxation activities, without the use of medication).

Patients, carers and all staff can all play a part in identifying the signs and symptoms of delirium. It is, in a sense, 'everybody's business'. Many things may contribute to someone's delirium, making it difficult to recognise and treat, but sometimes there may in fact be no obvious recognisable cause where a more detailed evaluation may indeed be necessary.

This topic is discussed fully in Chapter 3.

Common adverse outcomes

Delirium is strongly and independently associated with adverse outcomes.

The development of delirium in the hospital is associated with increased mortality rates, increased morbidity, functional decline, greater hospital costs, increased length of stay, and greater rates of care- or nursing-home placement. Poor outcomes are perhaps more likely in patients with severe and/or persistent delirium. This implies that aiming for reductions in both severity and duration of delirium are valid therapeutic goals. Knowledge of the underlying processes of the pathology of delirium may ultimately be the starting point for the development of novel orphan therapeutic interventions that have fewer adverse effects.

It should be noted the mechanisms underpinning associations between delirium and poor outcomes are currently rather unclear, specifically whether delirium has a direct aetiological role or serves as a marker for patients who will do poorly for a variety of other reasons. Both of these explanations may be true in any one individual in some circumstances.

This topic is discussed in greater detail in Chapter 8.

Wider differential diagnosis

Delirium is generally readily distinguished from other mental conditions because of its acute onset and fluctuating course. However, a clear informant history is not always available, and this needs to be borne in mind in any 'snapshot' assessment.

It is, however, worth noting that common differential diagnoses are dementia and depression. Distinguishing delirium from the neuropsychiatric symptoms of dementia can be daunting, but the context of disturbances (acute onset, fluctuating course, temporal relationship with an identifiable physical cause) and prominent problems in attention and arousal can point strongly towards delirium. Importantly, given the poor prognostic implications of delirium, it is safer to presume the diagnosis is delirium until otherwise established.

In order to differentiate between delirium and dementia, the most helpful factor is an account of the patient's pre-admission state from a relative or carer. This information is also relevant to the ultimate discharge of the patient from hospital. Serial measurements of cognition may help to differentiate delirium from dementia or detect its onset during a hospital admission.

Delirium symptoms can overlap with various psychiatric disorders, but in delirium disturbances of attention and other neuropsychological domains are more prominent.

Box 1.5 lists a possible wider differential diagnosis.

BOX 1.5 WIDER DIFFERENTIAL DIAGNOSIS

- Unipolar and bipolar depression
- Psychosis
- Catatonia (normal EEG; EEG needed to rule out non-status convulsive status; marked improvement with benzodiazepine test doses; behavioural system consisting of immobility/stupor, staring, mutism, posturing, rigidity, negativity, echolalia, echopraxia, stereotypies, rigidity, waxy flexibility)

- Malignant hyperthermia (pharmacogenetic disorder associated with inhalational anaesthetic exposure or a suxamethonium history after surgery; associated with skeletal muscle contractions)

- Neuroleptic malignant syndrome is a life-threatening syndrome, characterised by high fever, stiffness of the muscles, altered mental status and autonomic dysfunction. It has been associated with virtually all neuroleptics, including newer atypical antipsychotics, as well as a variety of other medications that affect central dopaminergic neurotransmission. Although originally described in patients receiving neuroleptic drugs, this syndrome may also occur in patients with Parkinson's disease who suddenly stop their L-dopa treatment.[67] It requires prompt recognition to prevent significant morbidity and death. Treatment includes immediately stopping the offending agent and implementing supportive measures including steps to lower the individual's body temperature. Complications are extremely serious.

- Serotonin syndrome. This is a clinical manifestation of excess serotonin in the central nervous system, resulting from the therapeutic use or overdose of serotonergic drugs, characterised by a triad of clinical features: neuromuscular excitation, autonomic effects and altered mental status. It is actually a spectrum of toxicity, ranging from mild to severe. The treatment of serotonin toxicity consists of ceasing the serotonergic medication, assessing the severity of toxicity, providing supportive care, and, in moderate and severe cases, the use of specific agents. Severe serotonin toxicity is a medical emergency that often requires emergency treatment.

- Central anticholinergic syndrome (dry submucous membranes; 'blind as a bat', 'mad as a hatter', 'red as a beet', 'dry as a bone', 'hot as a hare', 'stuffed as a pipe', seizures, tachycardia)

- Autoimmune encephalitis – may not be a typical delirium, subacute onset, rapid progression of short-term memory loss or working memory loss with new focal CNS findings including new-onset seizures, CSF pleiocytosis, MRI encephalitis. Treatment can include symptomatic and supportive treatments (including ECT, tumour removal and immune therapies).

Delirium as a syndrome of distress

Distress in delirium is common and often undetected, especially where there is no motor hyperactivity. However, patients often do not wish to volunteer this information readily. Proactive questioning about causative psychotic phenomena may be useful, and observation of the patient during the examination and informant history may provide additional information. If the patient is distressed, he should be examined for an obvious physical cause, pain (including gentle palpation of possible sites), urinary retention, distended abdomen, constipation and other potential sources of discomfort including even toothache. A 'pain instrument' to assess pain such as the **Abbey Pain Score**[68] might be used.

It is also important to provide a calm environment and frequent reassurance and explanation. Relatives should be involved where possible. One-to-one nursing can be helpful or, on the other hand, might contribute to the distress of a patient. Where safety permits, allowing a patient to move rather than be confined to a bed or a chair can reduce distress. The social model of disability reminds us that the problems experienced by a person are not simply due to being medically 'ill'. An approach to distress which is less biomedical and more humanistic, through perhaps the social model of disability, may be beneficial.[69] Individual distress might, in reframing, be associated with wider deep-seated oppressive behaviours and discrimination, and we need to acknowledge that 'the barriers that mental health service users face may sometimes be different, as well as similar, to those which people with physical, sensory and intellectual impairments face'.[70]

Clinicians who lack in-depth knowledge of delirium are more likely to view patients' behaviour as 'strange and incomprehensible', and might be unable to respond with the right level of care, support and empathy. At the carer level, there is a need for effective communication within the interprofessional team and between the interprofessional team and family carers, so that valuable observations and information are not lost. Because delirium is under-detected, carers are frequently left with no explanation from a healthcare professional as to why their loved one has had a profound change in their mental functioning. Carers often think that their relative has developed dementia or that a pre-existing dementia has suddenly 'accelerated'. It is thus very important not only to make the diagnosis formally and communicate this with the whole team but also to provide clear and consistent information to carers. This process can greatly be assisted by use of written materials such as the *Think Delirium* leaflet available from Healthcare Improvement Scotland.[71]

It may be fundamentally wrong to *assume* that patients experiencing hypoactive delirium experience little distress.

Signposting sources of support

Patients and carers both need support, which could come in a number of guises, including financial, emotional and informational. Quality improvement initiatives attempt to address this – see Chapter 12.

The management of delirium requires multidisciplinary approaches

Delirium is best managed by a multidisciplinary team, utilising comprehensive geriatric assessment in an appropriate environment with adequate staffing levels.

Delirium as a 'frailty syndrome'

Delirium and cognitive impairment in hospitals can be considered to be **frailty syndromes**. Frail older people are vulnerable to geriatric syndromes, and complications such as post-operative cognitive dysfunction and delirium. Frailty and delirium may, indeed, be different clinical expressions of a shared vulnerability to stress in older adults, and future research will determine what the precise cause of this vulnerability might be.[72]

A recent systematic review and meta-analysis (2018) supports the existence of an independent relationship between frailty and delirium, and future studies are needed to better delineate the dynamics between these syndromes in real time.[73] Frailty, which is a multifactorial syndrome manifested by a reduction in physiological reserve and in the ability to resist stressors, is a much more dynamic process than ageing alone.

Frailty is strongly related to delirium in older patients after discharge from the hospital.[74]

Although frailty and delirium are considered separate syndromes, they share common pathophysiological factors, including inflammation, atherosclerosis and malnutrition. A further relationship between the two syndromes is perhaps supported by the higher prevalence of frailty among individuals with delirium, and reports that frailty is associated with poorer functional outcomes and increased mortality in delirium.

Optimal perioperative care includes the identification of frailty, a multisystem and multidisciplinary evaluation preoperatively, and discussion of treatment goals and expectations. The **comprehensive geriatric assessment** can greatly help here.

The actual relationship between delirium and dementia

A growing body of evidence suggests that delirium can represent a pivotal life-changing event that is indicative of increased brain vulnerability, and can result in enhanced risk of persistent cognitive decline, including dementia.

Previous studies have documented that dementia is the leading risk factor for delirium, and delirium is an independent risk factor for subsequent dementia. However, a great deal of controversy surrounds whether delirium *needs* an underlying cognitive impairment to reveal itself.[75]

Delirium can unmask dementia pathology in cognitively normal or mildly impaired individuals, reducing time to dementia diagnoses.

In 2012, Davis and colleagues[76] confirmed that delirium is associated with general cognitive decline, an eightfold increase in incident dementia and accelerated decline in cognitive scores. The strong association with delirium, even after adjusting for age, in a general population reveals the significance of delirium in relation to dementia risk.

The importance of routinely referring patients with previous delirium to 'memory clinic' may therefore prove to be useful.

Prompt detection of dementia is critical to ensuring that persons having dementia and their carers have access to treatment, education, counselling and other post-diagnostic support services that can delay decline, prevent crises, ease carer burden and delay care-home placement.

Because delirium is partly preventable, delirium interventions might even prevent dementia. Delirium prevention offers opportunities for meaningful dementia prevention right now.[77]

DELPHIC

The Delirium and Population Health Informatics Cohort (DELPHIC) study is an observational population-based cohort study based in the London Borough of Camden. It is recruiting 2000 individuals aged 70 years and older and prospectively following them for two years, including daily ascertainment of all inpatient episodes for delirium.

The DELPHIC study represents an opportunity to characterise prospectively the impact of delirium on subsequent long-term cognitive impairment.

A definitive understanding of the natural history of delirium on risk of long-term cognitive impairment would have substantial implications for identification and follow-up of patients at high risk of dementia, targeting realistic therapeutic interventions and providing valid and prognostic information to patients and carers.

Differences between dementia and delirium

Delirium is not the same as dementia, which is chronic and generally irreversible.

Delirium is a sudden onset of change to the patient's baseline; they may become markedly more confused, withdrawn or agitated compared with their normal level of function. This can make it possible to distinguish delirium from dementia although it can be clinically challenging, and the two often co-exist. Dementia, on the other hand, causes a progressive decline in memory over a long period of time, usually months or years. Some types, such as dementia of Lewy bodies, can have symptoms similar to delirium including a fluctuating course and altered perception.

Cognitive decline after delirium may not simply be 'acceleration' of an underlying dementia pathological processes.[78] Identifying preventable factors that lead to neuronal injury in delirium, and strategies to target such factors, will be critical.

The issue of cognitive impairment in hospital, whether due to delirium, dementia or even something else, is fascinating, requires careful analysis, and is a very real issue:

> Undifferentiated cognitive impairment management includes treating patients as if they have delirium and possibly dementia. Unless the history is very clear, this should involve detailed characterisation of symptoms and impairments without necessarily giving a label, performed as part of comprehensive geriatric assessment. Therefore, management can be need driven, rather than diagnosis driven.[79]

A conceptual model has been proposed, synthesising how biomarker studies might advance our understanding of delirium and dementia, building on the concepts of vulnerability and resilience.[80]

Table 1.1 highlights the differences between dementia and delirium.

Table 1.1 A comparison of dementia and delirium

Clinical characteristics	Delirium	Dementia
Onset	Acute – subacute	Gradual – generally insidious
Course	Variable and hard to predict, fluctuating symptoms during the day, worsening at night	Gradual and long-lasting, symptoms are progressive and relatively stable over time
Progression	Sudden, unexpected	Slow but constant
Length	Hours, days, but rarely can be persistent	Months or years
Consciousness	Reduced	Clear
Vigilance and attention	Apathy or hypervigilance, fluctuating	Normal to diminished gross attention
Orientation	Generally much worsened, fluctuating in the most severe cases	Can worsen, especially in the advanced stages

cont.

Clinical characteristics	Delirium	Dementia
Memory	Short-term and immediate are worsened	Short-term and immediate are worsened; long-term memories often relatively spared
Thinking	Disorganised, distorted, fragmented, slowed down or accelerated	Difficult, repeated judgement, difficulty in finding the right words
Perception	Patients with delirium have specific visual perceptual deficits that cannot be accounted for by general cognitive impairment	Misperceptions, often absent
Motor behaviour	Variable, hypokinetic or hyperkinetic, or both	Normal, but there might be dyspraxia
Sleep–wake cycle	Altered with possible reversal of day and night	Fragmented but with possible reversal of day and night
Associated characteristics	Variable: emotional changes, exaggerations of personality, symptoms and signs of associated clinical conditions Speech and language disturbances are common	Attempts to hide intellectual deficits, personality changes, aphasia, agnosia, lack of comprehension
Mental status or performance in cognitive tasks	Distraction often sudden in onset	Progressively declining over a long period of time

The importance of quality improvement

Implementation science is the 'systematic study of how to design and evaluate a set of activities to facilitate successful uptake of an evidence-based health intervention'.[81] Many causal factors are described to impact implementation outcomes, such as patient, provider and organisational factors. Although patient-related risk factors account for a considerable part of the variability, they do not explain all of it.

Quality improvement is a framework to improve the way we work for the benefit of all patients and carers, and focuses on changing processes, not people.

With any product to implement, you have to decide whether to adopt it, adapt it or abandon it.

'Evidence-based' refers to 'interventions that have undergone sufficient scientific evaluation to be considered effective and/or are recommended by public health or professional organisations'.[82] From a research perspective, the collection of implementation science data is essential for programme evaluations and quality improvement.

This topic is considered in Chapter 12.

Electronic patient records

The digitalisation of healthcare for the purpose of medical documentation has led to huge amounts of data, which can be interpreted in numerous ways. Many healthcare events can be prevented when identified. 'Machine learning' algorithms could identify such events, but there is ambiguity in understanding the suggestions, especially in clinical setup. With an explosion of digital healthcare data, there is an opportunity to explore data and inherent health patterns.[83]

A main goal of health IT is to improve the quality and safety of patient care. Electronic health records (EHRs) can help patients receive optimal care by improving communication among providers, and promoting timely access to information at the point of care.

Endnotes

1   Barts Health NHS Trust (n.d.) 'Think Delirium.' Information card. Accessed on 28/11/2019 at www.dementiaaction.org.uk/assets/0002/1206/Think_Delirium_Cards.pdf.

2   Saxena, S. and Lawley, D. (2009) 'Delirium in the elderly: A clinical review.' *Postgraduate Medical Journal* 85, 1006, 405–413. Accessed on 28/11/2019 at www.ncbi.nlm.nih.gov/pubmed/19633006.

3   Siddiqi, N., House, A.O. and Holmes, J.D. (2006) 'Occurrence and outcome of delirium in medical in-patients: A systematic literature review.' *Age and Ageing 35*, 4, 350–364. Accessed on 28/11/2019 at www.ncbi.nlm.nih.gov/pubmed/16648149.

4   Slooter, A.J.C., Otte, W.M., Devlin, J.W., Arora, R.C. *et al.* (2020) 'Updated nomenclature of delirium and acute encephalopathy: Statement of ten Societies.' *Intensive Care Med.* Accessed on 24/02/2020 at https://doi.org/10.1007/s00134-019-05907-4.

5   Engel, G.L. and Romano, J. (1959) 'Delirium, a syndrome of cerebral insufficiency.' *Journal of Chronic Diseases 9*, 3, 260–277. Accessed on 28/11/2019 at www.ncbi.nlm.nih.gov/pubmed/13631039.

6   Mitchell, G. (2019) 'Undiagnosed delirium is common and difficult to predict among hospitalised patients.' *Evidence-Based Nursing.* doi: 10.1136/ebnurs-2019-103120. Accessed on 28/11/2019 at www.ncbi.nlm.nih.gov/pubmed/31296611.

7   Inouye, S.K. (2018) 'Delirium – A framework to improve acute care for older persons.' *Journal of the American Geriatrics Society 66*, 3, 446–451. Accessed on 28/11/2019 at www.ncbi.nlm.nih.gov/pubmed/29473940

8   Teodorczuk, A. and Billett, S. (2017) 'Mediating workplace situational pressures: The role of artefacts in promoting effective interprofessional work and learning.' *Focus on Health Professional Education 18*, 3. Accessed on 28/11/2019 at https://fohpe.org/FoHPE/article/view/158.

9   Morandi, A., Pozzi, C., Milisen, K., Hobbelen, H. *et al.* (2019) 'An interdisciplinary statement of scientific societies for the advancement of delirium care across Europe (EDA, EANS, EUGMS, COTEC, ITPOP/WCPT).' *BMC Geriatrics 19*, 253. Accessed on 28/11/2019 at https://bmcgeriatr.biomedcentral.com/articles/10.1186/s12877-019-1264-2.

10 Trzepacz, P.T., Baker, R.W. and Greenhouse, J. (1988) 'A symptom rating scale for delirium.' *Psychiatry Research 23*, 1, 89–97. Accessed on 28/11/2019 at www.sciencedirect.com/science/article/pii/0165178188900376?via%3Dihub.

11   Alosaimi, F.D., Alghamdi, A., Alsuhaibani, R., Alhammad, G. *et al.* (2018) 'Validation of the Stanford Proxy Test for Delirium (S-PTD) among critical and noncritical patients.' *Journal of Psychosomatic Research 114*, 8–14.

12   The 4AT is free to download at www.the4at.com.

13   Shenkin, S.D., Fox, C., Godfrey, M., Siddiqi, N. *et al.* (2019) 'Delirium detection in older acute medical inpatients: A multicentre prospective comparative diagnostic tests accuracy study of the 4AT and the confusion assessment method.' *BMC Medicine 17*, 138. Accessed on 28/11/2019 at https://bmcmedicine.biomedcentral.com/articles/10.1186/s12916-019-1367-9.

14   MacLullich, A.M., Shenkin, S.D., Goodacre, S., Godfrey, M. *et al.* (2019) 'The 4 "A"s test for detecting delirium in acute medical patients: A diagnostic accuracy study.' *Health Technology Assessment 23*, 40. Accessed on 28/11/2019 at www.journalslibrary.nihr.ac.uk/hta/hta23400/#/abstract.

15   Health Improvement Scotland (2019) *SIGN 157: Risk Reduction and Management of Delirium. A National Clinical Guideline.* Accessed on 28/11/2019 at www.sign.ac.uk/assets/sign157.pdf.

16   'F05: Delirium, not induced by alcohol and other psychoactive substances.' ICD-10 Version: 2014. Accessed on 13/12/2019 at https://icd.who.int/browse10/2014/en#!/F05.

17   Matar, E., Shine, J.M., Halliday, G.M. and Lewis, S.J.G. (2019) 'Cognitive fluctuations in Lewy body dementia: Towards a pathophysiological framework.' *Brain: A Journal of Neurology*, awz311. Accessed on 28/11/2019 at https://academic.oup.com/brain/advance-article-abstract/doi/10.1093/brain/awz311/5587662?redirectedFrom=fulltext.

18   Maldonado, J.R. (2018) 'Delirium pathophysiology: An updated hypothesis of the etiology of acute brain failure.' *International Journal of Geriatric Psychiatry 33*, 11, 1428–1457. Accessed on 28/11/2019 at www.ncbi.nlm.nih.gov/pubmed/29278283.

19   Mesulam, M.M. (2000) 'Attentional Networks, Confusional States and Neglect Syndromes.' In M.M. Mesulam (ed.) *Principles of Behavioural and Cognitive Neurology.* Oxford: Oxford University Press.

20   See e.g. www.1000livesplus.wales.nhs.uk/sitesplus/documents/1011/1000Lives%20poster%20%2D%202nd.pdf.

21   van Montford, S.J.T., van Dellen, E., Stam, C.J., Ahmad, A.H. *et al.* (2019) 'Brain network disintegration as a final common pathway for delirium: A systematic review and qualitative meta-analysis.' *NeuroImage: Clinical 23*, 101809. Accessed on 28/11/2019 at www.ncbi.nlm.nih.gov/pubmed/30981940.

22   Zipser, C.M., Knoepfel, S., Hayoz, P., Schubert, M. *et al.* (2019) 'Clinical management of delirium: The response depends on the subtypes. An observational cohort study in 602 patients.' *Palliative and Supportive Care*, 1–8, doi:10.1017/S1478951519000609. Accessed on 28/11/2019 at www.ncbi.nlm.nih.gov/pubmed/31506133.

23   American Psychiatric Association (2013) *Diagnostic and Statistical Manual of Mental Disorders, Fifth Edition (DSM-5).* Washington, DC: APA.

24   Yamada, C., Iwawaki, Y., Harada, K., Fukui, M., Morimoto, M. and Yamanaka, R. (2018) 'Frequency and risk factors for subsyndromal delirium in an intensive care unit.' *Intensive and Critical Care Nursing 47*, 15–22. Accessed on 28/11/2019 at www.ncbi.nlm.nih.gov/pubmed/29606481.

25   American Psychiatric Association (2013) *Diagnostic and Statistical Manual of Mental Disorders, Fifth Edition (DSM-5).* Washington, DC: APA.

26   Fick, D.M., Steis, M.R., Waller, J.L. and Inouye, S.K. (2013) 'Delirium superimposed on dementia is associated with prolonged length of stay and poor outcomes in hospitalized older adults.' *Journal of Hospital Medicine 8*, 9, 500–505. Accessed on 28/11/2019 at www.ncbi.nlm.nih.gov/pmc/articles/pmid/23955965.

27   Gore, R.L., Vardy, E.R.L.C. and O'Brien, J.T. (2015) 'Delirium and dementia with Lewy bodies: Distinct diagnoses or part of the same spectrum.' *Journal of Neurology, Neurosurgery, and Psychiatry 86*, 50–59. Accessed on 28/11/2019 at https://jnnp.bmj.com/content/86/1/50.

28   O'Dowd, S., Schumacher, J., Burn, D.J., Bonanni, L. *et al.* (2019) 'Fluctuating cognition in the Lewy body dementias.' *Brain 142*, 11, 3338–3350. Accessed on 28/11/2019 at https://academic.oup.com/brain/advance-article/doi/10.1093/brain/awz235/5549757.

29   McKeith, I.G., Perry, R.H., Fairbairn, A.F., Jabeen, S. and Perry, E.K. (1992) 'Operational criteria for senile dementia of Lewy body type (SDLT).' *Psychological Medicine 22*, 4, 911–922. Accessed on 28/11/2019 at www.ncbi.nlm.nih.gov/pubmed/1362617.

30   Bell, L.V. (1849) 'On a form of disease resembling some advanced stages of mania and fever, but so contradistinguished from any ordinary observed or described combination of symptoms as to render it probable that it may be overlooked and hitherto unrecorded malady.' *American Journal of Insanity 6*, 2, 97–127.

31 See e.g. Wetli, C.V. and Fishbain, D.A. (1985) 'Cocaine-induced psychosis and sudden death in recreational cocaine users.' *Journal of Forensic Sciences 30*, 3, 873–80; a good overview of this is given in Takeuchi, A., Ahern, T.L. and Henderson, S.O. (2011) 'Excited delirium.' *Western Journal of Emergency Medicine 12*, 1, 77–83. Accessed on 16/12/2019 at www.ncbi.nlm.nih.gov/pmc/articles/PMC3088378/#b1-wjem12_1p0077.

32 Kiely, D.K., Marcantonio, E.R., Inouye, S.K., Shaffer, M.L. *et al.* (2009) 'Persistent delirium predicts increased mortality.' *Journal of the American Geriatrics Society 57*, 1, 55–61. Accessed on 28/11/2019 at www.ncbi.nlm.nih.gov/pmc/articles/PMC2744464.

33 Cole, M.G., Ciampi, A., Belzile, E. and Zhong, L. (2009) 'Persistent delirium in older hospital patients: A systematic review of frequency and prognosis.' *Age and Ageing 38*, 1, 19–26. Accessed on 28/11/2019 at https://academic.oup.com/ageing/article/38/1/19/41354.

34 Silver, G., Traube, C., Gerber, L.M., Sun, X. *et al.* (2015) 'Pediatric delirium and associated risk factors: A single-center prospective observational study.' *Pedriatric Critical Care Medicine 16*, 4, 303–309. Accessed on 28/11/2019 at www.ncbi.nlm.nih.gov/pmc/articles/PMC5031497.

35 Traube, C., Mauer, E.A., Gerber, L.M., Kaur, S. *et al.* (2016) 'Cost associated with pediatric delirium in the intensive care unit.' *Critical Care Medicine 44*, 12, e1175–e1179. Accessed on 28/11/2019 at www.ncbi.nlm.nih.gov/pmc/articles/PMC5592112.

36 Trepacz, P.T. and Van der Mast, R.C. (2002) 'Pathophysiology of Delirium.' In J. Lindesay, K. Rockwood and A. Macdonald (eds) *Delirium in Old Age*. Oxford: Oxford University Press.

37 Massimo, L., Munoz, E., Hill, N., Mogle, J. *et al.* (2017) 'Genetic and environmental factors associated with delirium severity in older adults with dementia.' *International Journal of Geriatric Psychiatry 32*, 5, 574–581. Accessed on 28/11/2019 at www.ncbi.nlm.nih.gov/pubmed/27122004.

38 McCoy, T.H. Jr, Hart, K., Pellegrini, A. and Perlis, R.H. (2018) 'Genome-wide association identifies a novel locus for delirium risk.' *Neurobiology of Aging 68*, 160.e9–160.e14. Accessed on 28/11/2019 at www.ncbi.nlm.nih.gov/pmc/articles/PMC5993590.

39 van Munster, B.C., de Rooij, S.E. and Korevaar, J.C. (2009) 'The role of genetics in delirium in the elderly patient.' *Dementia and Geriatric Cognitive Disorders 28*, 3, 187–195. Accessed on 28/11/2019 at www.ncbi.nlm.nih.gov/pubmed/19713702.

40 Khan, B.A., Zawahiri, M., Campbell, N.L. and Boustani, M.A. (2013) 'Biomarkers for delirium – A review.' *Journal of the American Geriatrics Society 59*, 2, S256–S261. Accessed on 28/11/2019 at www.ncbi.nlm.nih.gov/pmc/articles/PMC3694326.

41 Nguyen, D.N., Huyghens, L., Zhang, H., Schiettecatte, J., Smitz, J. and Vincent, J.-L. (2014) 'Cortisol is an associated-risk factor of brain dysfunction in patients with severe sepsis and septic shock.' *BioMed Research International*, 712742. Accessed on 28/11/2019 at www.ncbi.nlm.nih.gov/pmc/articles/PMC4022165.

42 Chang, B.P. (2019) 'Can hospitalization be hazardous to your health? A nosocomial based stress model for hospitalization.' *General Hospital Psychiatry 60*, September–October, 83–89. Accessed on 28/11/2019 at www.sciencedirect.com/science/article/pii/S0163834319302282.

43 Maldonado, J.R. (2018) 'Delirium pathophysiology: An updated hypothesis of the etiology of acute brain failure.' *International Journal of Geriatric Psychiatry 33*, 11, 1428–1457. Accessed on 28/11/2019 at www.ncbi.nlm.nih.gov/pubmed/29278283.

44 Inouye, S.K. (2006) 'Delirium in older persons.' *New England Journal of Medicine 354*, 11, 1157–1165. Accessed on 28/11/2019 at www.ncbi.nlm.nih.gov/pubmed/16540616.

45 Marcantonio, E.R. (2017) 'Delirium in hospitalized older adults.' *New England Journal of Medicine 377*, 15, 1456–1466. Accessed on 28/11/2019 at www.ncbi.nlm.nih.gov/pmc/articles/PMC5706782.

46 Rowley-Conwy, G. (2017) 'Critical care nurses' knowledge and practice of delirium assessment.' *British Journal of Nursing 28*, 7. Accessed on 28/11/2019 at www.magonlinelibrary.com/doi/pdf/10.12968/bjon.2017.26.7.412.

47 Ravi, B., Pincus, D., Choi, S., Jenkinson, R., Wasserstein, D.N. and Redelmeier, D.A. (2019) 'Association of duration of surgery with postoperative delirium among patients receiving hip repair fracture.' *JAMA Network Open 2*, 2, e190111. Accessed on 28/11/2019 at https://jamanetwork.com/journals/jamanetworkopen/fullarticle/2725493.

48 Australian Commission on Safety and Quality in Health Care (2018) 'Hospital-acquired complications (HACs).' Accessed on 28/11/2019 at www.safetyandquality.gov.au/our-work/indicators/hospital-acquired-complications.

49   Saunders, R., Seaman, K., Graham, R. and Christiansen, A. (2019) 'The effect of volunteers' care and support on the health outcomes of older adults in acute care: A systematic scoping review.' *Journal of Clinical Nursing 28*, 23–24, 4236–4249. Accessed on 28/11, 2019 at www.ncbi.nlm.nih.gov/pubmed/31429987.

50   Rockwood, K., Lindsay, M.K.W. and Davis, D.H. (2019) 'Genetic predisposition and modifiable risks for late-life dementia.' *Nature Medicine 25*, 1331–1332. Accessed on 28/11/2019 at www.nature.com/articles/s41591-019-0575-3.

51   Zipser, C.M., Deuel, J., Ernst, J., Schubert, M. *et al.* (2019) 'Predisposing and precipitating factors for delirium in neurology: A prospective cohort study of 1487 patients.' *Journal of Neurology 266*, 12, 3065–3075. Accessed on 28/11/2019 at www.ncbi.nlm.nih.gov/pubmed/31520105.

52   Magny, E., Le Petitcorps, H., Pociumban, M., Bouksani-Kacher, Z. *et al.* (2018) 'Predisposing and precipitating factors for delirium in community-dwelling older adults admitted to hospital with this condition: A prospective case series.' *PLOS One 13*, 2, e0193034. Accessed on 29/11/2019 at www.ncbi.nlm.nih.gov/pmc/articles/PMC5825033.

53   Hayden, E.Y., Putman, J., Nunez, S., Shin, W.S. *et al.* (2019) 'Ischemic axonal injury up-regulates MARK4 in cortical neurons and primes tau phosphorylation and aggregation.' *Acta Neuropathologica Communications 7*, 1, 135. Accessed on 29/11/2019 at www.ncbi.nlm.nih.gov/pubmed/31429800.

54   Goto, T., Yoshida, K., Tsugawa, Y., Camargo, C.A., Jr, and Hasegawa K. (2016) 'Infectious disease-related emergency department visits of elderly adults in the United States, 2011–2012.' *Journal of the American Geriatrics Society 64*, 1, 31–36. Accessed on 16/12/2019 at www.ncbi.nlm.nih.gov/pubmed/26696501.

55   Smith, M.-A., Puckrin, R., Lam, P.W., Lamb, M.J., Simor, A.E. and Leis, J.A. (2019) 'Association of increased colony-count threshold for urinary pathogens in hospitalized patients with antimicrobial treatment.' *JAMA Internal Medicine 179*, 7, 990–992. Accessed on 29/11/2019 at https://jamanetwork.com/journals/jamainternalmedicine/fullarticle/2731706.

56   Balogun, S.A. and Philbrick, J.T. (2014) 'Delirium, a symptom of UTI in the elderly: Fact or fable? A systematic review.' *Canadian Geriatrics Journal 17*, 1, 22–26. Accessed on 29/11/2019 at www.ncbi.nlm.nih.gov/pmc/articles/PMC3940475.

57   Teale, E.A., Munyombwe, T., Schuurmans, M., Siddiqi, N., and Young, J. (2018) 'A prospective study to investigate utility of the Delirium Observational Screening Scale (DOSS) to detect delirium in care home residents.' *Age and Ageing 47*, 1, 56–61. Accessed on 29/11/2019 at http://eprints.whiterose.ac.uk/119038/3/DOSS%20primary%20paper_final%20manuscript_author%20accepted%20version.pdf.

58   e.g. Ding, Y., Niu, J., Zhang, Y., Liu, W. *et al.* (2018) 'Informant questionnaire on cognitive decline in the elderly (IQCODE) for assessing the severity of dementia in patients with Alzheimer's disease.' *BMC Geriatrics 18*, 136. Accessed on 29/11/2019 at https://bmcgeriatr.biomedcentral.com/articles/10.1186/s12877-018-0837-9.

59   DiBattista, A.M., Heinsinger, N.M. and Rebeck, G.W. (2016) 'Alzheimer's disease genetic risk factor APOE4 also affects normal brain function.' *Current Alzheimer Research 13*, 11, 1200–1207. Accessed on 29/11/2019 at www.ncbi.nlm.nih.gov/pmc/articles/PMC5839141.

60   Hong, N. and Park, J.-Y. (2018) 'The motoric types of delirium and estimated blood loss during perioperative period in orthopedic elderly patients.' *BioMed Research International*, 9812041. Accessed on 29/11/2019 at www.ncbi.nlm.nih.gov/pmc/articles/PMC6236653.

61   Janssen, T.L., Alberts, A.R., Hooft, L., Mattace-Raso, F.U.S., Mosk, C.A. and van der Laan, L. (2019) 'Prevention of postoperative delirium in elderly patients planned for elective surgery: Systematic review and meta-analysis.' *Clinical Interventions in Aging 14*, 1095–1117. Accessed on 29/11/2019 at www.ncbi.nlm.nih.gov/pmc/articles/PMC6590846.

62   van Velthuijsen, E.L., Zwakhalen, S.M.G., Pijpers, E., van de Ven, L.I. *et al.* (2018) 'Effects of a medication review on delirium in older hospitalised patients: A comparative retrospective cohort study.' *Drugs and Aging 35*, 2, 153–161. Accessed on 29/11/2019 at www.ncbi.nlm.nih.gov/pmc/articles/PMC5847150/#CR10.

63   Milisen, K., Lemiengre, J., Braes, T. and Foreman, M.D. (2005) 'Multicomponent intervention strategies for managing delirium in hospitalized older people: Systematic review.' *Journal of Advanced Nursing 52*, 1, 79–90. Accessed on 29/11/2019 at www.ncbi.nlm.nih.gov/pubmed/16149984.

64   'Disease prevention.' nature.com. Accessed on 16/12/2019 at www.nature.com/subjects/disease-prevention.

65   Hodes, J.F., Oakley, C.I., O'Keefe, J.H., Lu, P. *et al.* 'Alzheimer's "prevention" vs. "risk reduction": Transcending semantics for clinical practice.' *Frontiers in Neurology 9*, 1179. Accessed on 29/11/2019 at www.frontiersin.org/articles/10.3389/fneur.2018.01179/full.

66   Hospital Elder Life Program (HELP) for Prevention of Delirium: https://hospitalelderlifeprogram.org.

67   Serrano-Dueñas, M. (2003) 'Neuroleptic malignant syndrome-like, or–dopaminergic malignant syndrome–due to levodopa therapy withdrawal. Clinical features in 11 patients.' *Parkinsonism & Related Disorders, 9,* 3, 175–817. Accessed on 24/02/2020 at https://doi.org/10.1016/S1353-8020(02)00035-4.

68   See www.mdcalc.com/abbey-pain-scale-dementia-patients.

69   Beresford, P. (n.d.) 'Disability, Distress and New Thinking.' Sage Video Tutorials. Accessed on 29/11/2019 at http://sk.sagepub.com/video/skpromo/9llLu8/disability-distress-and-new-thinking.

70   Beresford, P. *et al.* (2010) 'Towards a social model of madness and distress? Exploring what service users say.' Joseph Rowntree Foundation. Accessed on 29/11/2019 at www.jrf.org.uk/report/towards-social-model-madness-and-distress-exploring-what-service-users-say.

71   NHS Tayside, in collaboration with Healthcare Improvement Scotland and NHS boards (2018) 'Think Delirium: Information for patient, families and carers.' Accessed 17/02/2020 at https://tinyurl.com/rlbnru3.

72   Quinlan, N., Marcantonio, E.R., Inouye, S.K., Gill, T.M., Kamholz, B. and Rudolph, J.L. (2011) 'Vulnerability: The crossroads of frailty and delirium.' *Journal of the American Geriatrics Society 59,* Suppl. 2, S262–2268. Accessed on 29/11/2019 at www.ncbi.nlm.nih.gov/pubmed/22091571.

73   Perisco, I., Cesari, M., Morandi, A., Haas, J. *et al.* (2018) 'Frailty and delirium in older adults: A systematic review and meta-analysis of the literature.' *Journal of the American Geriatrics Society 66,* 10, 2022–2030. Accessed on 29/11/2019 at www.ncbi.nlm.nih.gov/pubmed/30238970.

74   Verloo, H., Goulet, C., Morin, D. and von Gunten, A. (2016) 'Association between frailty and delirium in older adult patients discharged from hospital.' *Clinical Interventions in Aging 11,* 55–63. Accessed on 29/11/2019 at www.ncbi.nlm.nih.gov/pmc/articles/PMC4723030.

75   Fong, T.G., Davis, D., Growdon, M.E., Albuquerque, A. and Inouye, S.K. (2015) 'The interface of delirium and dementia in older persons.' *Lancet Neurology 14,* 8, 823–832. Accessed on 29/11/2019 at www.ncbi.nlm.nih.gov/pmc/articles/PMC4535349.

76   Davis, D.H., Muniz Terrera, G., Keage, H., Rahkonen, T. *et al.* (2012) 'Delirium is a strong risk factor for dementia in the oldest-old: A population-based cohort study.' *Brain: A Journal of Neurology 135,* 9, 2809–2916. Accessed on 29/11/2019 at www.ncbi.nlm.nih.gov/pubmed/22879644.

77   Hayden, K.M., Inouye, S.K., Cunningham, C., Jones, R.N. *et al.* (2018) 'Reduce the burden of dementia now.' *Alzheimer's and Dementia 14,* 7, 845–847. Accessed on 29/11/2019 at www.ncbi.nlm.nih.gov/pubmed/29959910.

78   Fong, T.G., Inouye, S.K. and Jones, R.N. (2017) 'Delirium, dementia, and decline.' *JAMA Psychiatry 74,* 3, 212–213. Accessed on 29/11/2019 at https://jamanetwork.com/journals/jamapsychiatry/fullarticle/2598160.

79   Jackson, T.A., Gladman, J.R.F., Harwood, R.H., MacLullich, A.M.J. *et al.* (2017) 'Challenges and opportunities in understanding dementia and delirium in the acute hospital.' *PLOS Medicine 14,* 3, e1002247. Accessed on 29/11/2019 at https://journals.plos.org/plosmedicine/article?id=10.1371/journal.pmed.1002247

80   Fong, T.G., Vasunilashorn, S.M., Libermann, T., Marcantonio, E.R. and Inouye, S.K. (2019) 'Delirium and Alzheimer disease: A proposed model for shared pathophysiology.' *International Journal of Geriatric Psychiatry 34,* 6, 781–789. Accessed on 29/11/2019 at www.ncbi.nlm.nih.gov/pubmed/30773695.

81   Handley, M.A., Gorukanti, A. and Cattamanchi, A. (2015) 'Strategies for implementing implementation science: A methodological overview.' *Emergency Medicine Journal 33,* 9. Accessed on 29/11/2019 at https://emj.bmj.com/content/33/9/660.

82   Handley, M.A., Gorukanti, A. and Cattamanchi, A. (2015) 'Strategies for implementing implementation science: A methodological overview.' *Emergency Medicine Journal 33,* 9. Accessed on 29/11/2019 at https://emj.bmj.com/content/33/9/660.

83   Veeranki, S.P.K., Hayn, D., Jauk, S., Quehenberger, F. *et al.* (2019) 'An improvised classification model for predicting delirium.' *Studies in Health Technology and Informatics 264,* 1566–1567. Accessed on 29/11/2019 at www.ncbi.nlm.nih.gov/pubmed/31438234.

2

Delirium identification, assessment and diagnosis

LEARNING OBJECTIVES

In this chapter, you will be able to consider in much greater detail the content and style of the approach you could use in identifying, assessing and diagnosing delirium and its subtypes.

Overview

Partly because it is frequently missed in routine clinical care, delirium is associated with poor outcomes. Delirium is a clinical condition based on validated criteria and consensus definitions, such as the DSM or ICD criteria. But the nature of the 'core symptoms' continues to be debated. Further epidemiological work is suggested here.

An astute clinician will probably be able to identify without much difficulty a primary cause but should nonetheless still be aware of multiple contributors to the clinical syndrome under consideration in a given patient. Multiple causes of delirium occur particularly in the elderly. Specific management of delirium is of obvious and immediate benefit to patients in many clinical situations.

The need for 'short screening instruments'

Examples of short screening tests are given below in Table 2.1.

Any management response has to be appropriate for the screening to be of any value.

Most attention tests used in the assessment of delirium are sensitive to delirium. This may be because lower levels of attention, notably sustained attention and orienting, are a prerequisite for higher levels of attentional and cognitive functioning. Vigilance tests provide a relatively 'pure' measure of attention, whereas backward span tests and 'months of the year backwards' (MOYTB) measure multiple cognitive domains. There is some evidence supporting the view that sustained attention is disproportionately affected in delirium.

Table 2.1 Short screening tests

Name of test	Comment
6-CIT	The 6-CIT measures attention, temporal orientation and short-term memory. It is scored out of 28, with higher scores indicating greater degree of impairment. It is an exclusively verbal test, hence can be used in those with visual or fine motor impairments.
UB-2	The Ultra-Brief 2-Item Screener is a clinician-administered two-item interview designed for large-scale delirium case identification. The two items are 'Please tell me the day of the week' and 'Please tell me the months of the year backwards; say December as your first month'.
Spatial span forwards	Spatial span forwards can be performed using a white card with squares evenly spaced over three rows. Predetermined sequences of squares are tapped out for the patient to repeat, beginning with a sequence of two and up to a maximum of seven. A cut-off of 4/5 has been suggested.
Months of the year backwards (MOYTB)	MOYTB can be scored in several ways; however, there is no consensus as to which is actually best. Subjects are invited to say the months forward from January and subsequently asked to recite them backwards from December.

A patient must be arousable to voice in order to assess for delirium. Thus, an arousal/sedation tool must be utilised along with a delirium assessment tool. The **Richmond Agitation Sedation Scale** is an assessment tool that was originally designed to assess sedation and agitation on a continuous numerical scale (−5 to +4) in intensive care. It can be administered in ten seconds and is largely observational. In contrast to arousal tests, cognitive tests may be impacted by patient factors such as dysphasia, illness severity, drowsiness, fatigue and severe deafness, which may limit their applicability and may be low in dementia in the absence of delirium.

Cognitive tests can elicit a quantitative measure of the *type* and *extent* of deficit which can be compared over time. Patients may not tolerate repeated demands to perform such tests, however. The introduction of clear diagnostic criteria for delirium has supported considerable growth in research activity in the field of delirium. The essential criteria have been progressively abbreviated, and studies indicate considerable disparity in delirium detection when applying different DSM versions and ICD-10.

Evidence underlying evaluation of common tools such as CAM and 4AT

An **ideal screening tool for delirium** should be brief, specific, sensitive, inexpensive, require little or no training and be appropriate to the clinical setting it is being applied to. It should reliably detect those with delirium and also have acceptable specificity, accurately identifying those without delirium as screen negative. Assessment is the cornerstone to effective, person-centred patient care. It is a regulatory requirement that registered professionals can accurately assess all patients of normal or worsening condition.

Recommended practice suggests that patients should be assessed by observation a few times daily for changes in behaviour which might indicate delirium. Doing so might detect behavioural changes early enough to prevent the onset of delirium in the first instance. It is felt that the objective accuracy of health professionals in diagnosing delirium without the use of a screening tool has been inadequate.

Nurses, who spend more time at the bedside than physicians, play a crucial role in the recognition of delirium. They have regular contact with patients, assuming no obstructive system issues such as 'rota gaps', and are better able to observe fluctuations in attention, level of consciousness and cognitive functioning. As a result, observations made by nurses are critical for the early detection and management of delirium.

Two factors have been linked to delirium that is undetected by nurses among elderly hospitalised patients: its *forms* and its *fluctuating nature*.[1] The fluctuation of symptoms during the course of the day that is characteristic of episodes of delirium make the identification of delirium problematic. Delirium may go undetected if the evaluation is not based on observations gathered over a sufficiently long period of time.

The Confusion Assessment Method

The **Confusion Assessment Method** (CAM) was originally developed in 1988–1990 to improve the identification and recognition of delirium.

The CAM is included in multiple guidelines and policy documents, and has been translated into more than 20 languages. It has been validated in both research and clinical settings and consists of a rating system based on nine features (acute onset, inattention, disorganised thinking, altered level of consciousness, disorientation, memory impairment, perceptual disturbances, psychomotor agitation or retardation, and altered sleep–wake cycle) operationalised from the DSM and a briefer diagnostic algorithm used for screening.

When validated against the reference standard ratings of geriatric psychiatrists based on comprehensive psychiatric assessment, the CAM had a sensitivity of 94–100%, specificity of 90–95%, and high inter-observer reliability in the original study.[2] More recently, this work has been extended in seven high-quality validation studies on over a thousand subjects, where the CAM had a sensitivity of 94% and specificity of 89%.[3]

Some means of cognitive testing, such as the Mini-Cog or SQPMSQ, is recommended in order to score the CAM. These tests are not lengthy and can be completed in a matter of minutes.

The scoring of CAM is shown in Figure 2.1.

---

(1) acute onset and fluctuating course
and
(2) inattention
and either
(3) disorganized thinking
or
(4) altered level of consciousness

[Scored based on cognitive testing. See details at www.hospitalelderlifeprogram.org]

Figure 2.1 Scoring of CAM[4]

Reproduced with kind permission of Prof. Sharon Inouye.

'CAM-positive delirium' requires the presence of 1 and 2 and either 3 or 4.

Because of the need for a bedside interview and brief cognitive test before scoring, it generally takes about 5–7 minutes to complete. Additional tools have been created from the original test including the 3D CAM[5] and Family-CAM (FAM-CAM)[6] instruments. The 3D-CAM can be completed in an average of three minutes and performs very well compared with an expert evaluator. The FAM-CAM may be administered to a family caregiver by phone or in person, or can be self-administered, allowing for delirium assessment in a wide range of settings.

The CAM is recommended in multiple care pathways and incorporated into electronic medical record (EMR) systems around the world.

4AT

The **4AT** is a sensitive method of screening for delirium in hospitalised older people; ongoing research in validation meta-analysis demonstrates its high specificity too. Its brevity and simplicity make it well suited for routine clinical practice, and the instrument has been validated in culturally diverse geriatric inpatients including the acute medical setting, making it a suitable screening tool for a geriatric patient population. The 4AT not only performs well in studies, but can be successfully implemented in electronic care records. There is, however, scope for further research in the use of 4AT in settings such as residential homes.

Currently the 4AT is widely used internationally in the UK, many European countries and Australasia, and has rapidly increasing use globally.

It allows for assessment of 'untestable' patients (those who cannot undergo cognitive testing or interview because of severe drowsiness or agitation). Some studies have recommended the 4AT over CAM as it is less open to interpretation, has a higher sensitivity[7] and is quicker to use. The 4AT is also supported as the assessment tool of choice by older emergency department attendees.

Other screening tools

Other tools generally have significant disadvantages over CAM and 4AT, such as longer assessment time, poorer sensitivity and/or specificity, and/or relative lack of validation.

The 13-item **Delirium Observation Screening Scale** has good specificity and sensitivity but requires assessment over three shift periods; its authors have suggested it is geared more towards detection of hyperactive delirium.[8]

Other screening tools include a 16-item Delirium Rating Scale, Memorial Delirium Assessment Scale, and Delirium Symptom Interview. Since the severity of delirium is also an important outcome predictor, quantifying the severity is useful to guide clinical management. These scales include CAM-S (severity) long and short forms, Confusion Rating Scale, Delirium Assessment Scale and Delirium Rating Scale.

DSM and ICD

The diagnosis of delirium is based on clinical assessment and is guided by standardised criteria. The delirium diagnostic criteria of the *International Classification of Diseases*, tenth edition (ICD-10)[9] and the recently published *Diagnostic Statistical Manual of Mental Disorders*, fifth edition (DSM-5)[10] represent definitive standards in terms of diagnosis, based on the best available evidence and maximal expert consensus at the time of their publication.

Earlier studies comparing the delirium diagnostic criteria of DSM-IV and ICD-10 suggest that the DSM criteria were more inclusive. In research studies, use of either ICD-10 or DSM-5 criteria is recommended as the 'gold standard' diagnostic criteria.

The relevance of protocols

At an institutional level, policies, protocols and guidelines regarding delirium detection need to be developed and implemented, and supported by effective and appropriate educational initiatives. The implementation of guidelines on delirium recognition and screening is facilitated by many factors including leadership, promotion as a quality improvement and safety culture initiative, and electronic health record documentation.

It appears advisable to improve clinical documentation by developing screening tools that can be easily integrated into the electronic medical record, which the whole team can access. Specifically, baseline cognitive function and delirium measurements need to be integrated into updated electronic medical record systems.

Educational initiatives are discussed in Chapter 13.

The importance of cognitive assessment of older people in the emergency department

Some countries use financial incentives to encourage cognitive screening at the point of hospital admission. Validated, short cognitive screening tools could allow emergency department (ED) staff to identify older attendees with cognitive vulnerability, triggering appropriate care pathways and urgent assessment of those with possible delirium.

Cognitive impairment is a frequent problem among older patients attending the ED and can be the result of pre-existing cognitive impairment, delirium or neurological disorders. Another cause can also be acute disturbance of brain perfusion and oxygenation, which may be reversed by optimal resuscitation. In the recent APOP study (2019), abnormal vital signs were associated with decreased brain perfusion and oxygenation and are also associated with cognitive impairment in older ED patients.[11]

A **lack of screening of delirium** in the ED may be accounted for by the following:

- the perceived difficulty using a delirium screening tool

- screening being excessively time-consuming in a busy clinical environment

- negative beliefs about older people such as assuming that mental confusion is normal in older adults

- system-level limitations including time constraints in care provision and frequent staff turnover

- lack of feasible delirium assessments available for the dynamic ED environment.

Essential role of the multidisciplinary team working in the assessment of delirium

Senior doctors and nurses should ensure that doctors-in-training and nurses are able to recognise and treat delirium. The approaches might involve more than one professional discipline. There is an important difference between the terms 'multidisciplinary' and 'interdisciplinary'.[12]

- In *multidisciplinary* teams, the patient is assessed individually by several professionals. Participants may have separate but interrelated roles, but observe their own disciplinary boundaries.

- In *interdisciplinary* teams, members come together as a whole to discuss their individual assessments and develop a plan for the patient. Teams integrate closer to complete a 'shared goal'.

Liaison psychiatry services have a valuable role in preventing and managing delirium. In particular, help should be sought if there are behavioural problems. Many patients with delirium have an underlying long-term cognitive impairment which may be best followed up and managed by a psychiatrist of old age.

As with all elderly patients, discharge should be planned in conjunction with all disciplines involved in caring for the patient, both in hospital and in the community (including informal carers).

Practical arrangements should be in place prior to discharge for activities such as washing, dressing and medication.

Important clinical symptoms

It is important to assess some key clinical aspects to delirium.

Wandering

Wandering itself is potentially an unnecessarily pejorative term, but in patients experiencing delirium it can be a genuine phenomenon reflecting inattention, poor memory, anxiety and distractibility. Patients who 'wander' may require close observation within a safe and reasonably closed environment, but human rights considerations are nevertheless paramount (Chapter 10).

The least restrictive option should always be used when acting in the best interests of the patient to keep them safe from assessed risk.

In the first instance, attempts should be made to identify and remedy possible causes of anxiety or agitation, such as pain, thirst, need for a toilet, a perceived threat to personal security or safety. The use of restraints or sedation should only be used as a final option, once others have been tried, and only if they can be justified as being in the best interests of the patient.

Sedation

Keep the use of sedatives and major tranquillisers to a minimum. The main aim of drug treatment is the treatment of distressing or dangerous behavioural disturbance (e.g. agitation and hallucinations).

Excited delirium syndrome

As **excited delirium syndrome** (ExDS) does not currently have a known specific aetiology or a consistent single anatomical feature, it can only be described by its epidemiology, commonly described clinical presentation and usual course. Historically, in ExDS there is typically a component of illicit drug use or underlying psychiatry such as schizophrenia.

Differential diagnosis

The general public, law enforcement and even highly trained medical personnel will not be readily able to readily discern the cause of an acute behavioural disturbance, or differentiate a specific organic disease from ExDS based solely on observation. Almost any drug, toxin, extraneous substance, psychiatric or medical condition, or biochemical or physiological alteration in the body can cause acute changes in behaviour or mental status.

Several specific entities that cause altered mental status and may mimic

ExDS deserve specific mention. However, they usually do not share the aggressive violent behaviour manifested by patients with ExDS.

Examples include the following:

- diabetic hypoglycaemic reactions, associated with irritability, shakiness, sweatiness and dizziness

- 'heat stroke', manifested as tactile hyperthermia, rhabdomyolysis and delirium, and may be associated with neuroleptic use and mental illness

- thyrotoxicosis, manifested in a similar clinical presentation, especially during episodes of a 'thyroid storm'

- serotonin syndrome and neuroleptic malignant syndrome – may share some clinical characteristics with ExDS.

Certain psychiatric syndromes may mimic ExDS. Some patients experience behavioural disturbances directly due to psychotropic drug withdrawal or non-compliance. Substance abuse is also very common in psychiatric patients. Many psychiatric conditions themselves, including acute paranoid schizophrenia, bipolar disorder and acute stressful reactions, may mimic an ExDS-like state.

The legal implications of this important condition are considered more in Chapter 10.

Common subtypes of delirium

This topic was first introduced in Chapter 1.

Hyperactive delirium is where a patient is likely to be restless, experience distressing hallucinations and delusions, and display socially inappropriate behaviours which are typically more easily recognised. It is a less common form of delirium. Irrelevant stimuli can startle the patient easily.[13]

Delusions are typically fleeting, often persecutory and usually related to the disorientation. Visual hallucinations are characteristic and strongly suggest delirium. However, hallucinations in auditory and other sensory modalities can also occur.

In 2000, Meagher and Trzepacz[14] found that delusions, hallucinations, mood changes, speech disturbances and sleep disturbances are more frequent in hyperactive patients. It is recognised that the 'waxing and waning' nature of the symptoms and sleep–wake cycle abnormalities also impedes our understanding.

Hypoactive delirium is characterised by slowed cognition, lethargy and visible sleepiness, and decreased movement. It is found more commonly in the elderly, with age >65 years being an independent risk factor. This is the more common form of delirium and is often misdiagnosed as depression; it also carries the greater mortality risk.

It typically requires active screening with delirium assessment tools to diagnose since it is often less clinically apparent than the restlessness and agitated behaviour of hyperactive delirium. Hypoactive delirium is often missed as the patient may be somnolent, inactive and wake up from anaesthetic quietly.

Mixed delirium is a combination of hyperactive and hypoactive delirium, where a person may fluctuate between signs and symptoms of the two. These signs and symptoms are not exclusive to a delirium diagnosis and thus present a diagnostic issue.

Why an early diagnosis of delirium is important and the likely outcomes if assessment and treatment is delayed

'Think delirium'[15] is a policy created in line with the most recent recommended clinical guidelines which promotes the rapid diagnosis and effective treatment of an episode of delirium. If delirium is effectively identified and treated, significant financial and human cost could be saved.

An unfortunate barrier to delirium assessment is the wide variety of detection tools available. This to some extent reflects the clinical heterogeneity of the condition and the varying skills of assessors, with identification of some cases of delirium made through observed behaviours and other cases by detailed cognitive assessment requiring more expertise. The use of delirium assessment tools in research studies may differ from its implementation in the clinical environment.

Regular mental status assessment needs to become a 'vital sign' embedded into basic hospital care. One important advance in the UK is the adoption of a new **National Early Warning Score** (NEWS), which incorporates a four-point level of consciousness measure. The NEWS score has been developed in part to pick up 'new-onset or worsening confusion, delirium or any other altered mentation [which] should always prompt concern about potentially serious underlying causes and warrants urgent clinical evaluation.'[16]

Some recent evidence suggests that the reduced level of consciousness is a specific (though not sensitive) sign of delirium, and so it could become a stimulus for specific delirium screening, bolstering rates of detection. These and other and 'system-wide approaches', embedded into routine practice, are likely required to address the huge unmet need for delirium assessment.

Identification of the presenting issues in delirium

The main developing problems in delirium are:

- falls

- pressure sores

- nosocomial infections

- functional impairment

- continence problems

- over-sedation

- malnutrition

- restraints that have not been shown to prevent falls and may indeed increase the risk of injury.

It may be preferable to nurse the patient on a low bed or place the mattress directly on the floor. Adoption of the good practices described should make the use of physical restraints unnecessary for the management of confusion. Some important aspects are:

- **Pressure sores:** Patients should have a formal pressure sore risk assessment (e.g. Norton score or Waterlow score) and receive regular pressure area care, including special mattresses where necessary. Patients should be mobilised as soon as their illness allows.

- **Functional impairment:** Assessment by a therapist to maintain and improve functional ability should be considered in all patients experiencing delirium.

- **Continence:** A full continence assessment should be carried out. Regular toileting and prompt treatment of urinary tract infections may prevent urinary incontinence. Catheters should be avoided where possible because of the increased risks of trauma and the risk of catheter-associated infection.

- **Malnutrition:** It is often difficult for delirium patients to eat enough to meet increased metabolic needs. Food alternatives should take into account the patient's preferences. Adequate staffing levels should be ensured to provide support, personalised if necessary, to encourage eating. Oral nutritional supplements can be considered.

Assessment

Consider acute, life-threatening conditions, including low oxygen level, low blood pressure, low glucose level, and drug intoxication or withdrawal.

Systematically identify and treat potential causes (medications, acute illness, etc.), noting that multiple causes are common.

History

Many patients with delirium are unable to provide an accurate history. Wherever possible, **corroboration** should be sought from the carer, general practitioner or any source with good knowledge of patients experiencing delirium.

Acute triggers of delirium commonly include infection, dehydration, severe constipation, urinary retention, pain, critical illness, surgery (especially heart and hip operations) and side effects of new medicines or medicine withdrawal.

In addition to standard questions in the history, the following information should be specifically sought, itemised in Box 2.1.

BOX 2.1 SOME FEATURES OF A DETAILED HISTORY

- Onset and course of confusion
- Previous cognition
- Full drug history including non-prescribed drugs and recent drug cessation
- Alcohol and other drug history
- Functional activities of daily living (ADLs)
- History of diet and food intake
- History of bladder and bowel voiding
- Previous episodes of acute or chronic confusion
- Symptoms suggestive of underlying cause
- Sensory deficits
- Any sensory aids used
- Pre-admission social circumstances – especially mobility – and any existent care package
- Comorbid illness

Communication between people from different disciplines is essential to avoid unnecessary repetition of information gathering.

Examination

A full physical examination should be carried out.

Physical examination is highly effective for the physician and can aid with narrowing the differential diagnosis. Examination might be challenging because of patients' agitation or uncooperativeness or, conversely, hypersomnolence.

Physicians should pay attention to the following, shown in Box 2.2.

BOX 2.2 EXAMINATION

General

- Nutritional status (general observations and MUST score[17]).
- Evidence of pyrexia.
- Search for infection: lungs, urine, abdomen, skin.
- Evidence of alcohol abuse or other drug withdrawal.

Head, eyes, ears, nose, throat

- It is important to examine the head, as it can show signs of trauma.
- Poorly reactive pupils may suggest cerebral herniation.
- Exophthalmos may indicate underlying thyroid pathology.
- Eye examination can also give a clue as to the existence of toxicology (miosis, mydriasis, nystagmus).
- Ophthalmoplegia could suggest Wernicke encephalopathy in the appropriate clinical setting. Vertical nystagmus can be a sign of intracranial process or phencyclidine ingestion, while rotary nystagmus can be a sign of ingestion of a drug of abuse such as phencyclidine.[18]

Neck

- Examination of the neck provides information about meningism and goitre.

Cardiovascular

- New murmur can be seen in infective endocarditis, which in turn can cause sepsis and delirium.

Respiratory

- Abnormal lung sounds can suggest pneumonia.

Skin

- Skin examination might reveal a diaphoresis as seen in overdose from sympathomimetics. Rashes or purpura can be seen in meningococcal septicaemia.

Musculoskeletal

- Consider muscular examination, as it could reveal lead-pipe rigidity as can be seen in neuroleptic malignant syndrome.

Neurological

- Note patient's GCS (Glasgow Coma Scale)/AVPU (an acronym from 'alert, verbal, pain, unresponsive) and check for focal neurological deficits suggesting intracranial pathology.

Assessment of speech

- Cognitive function using a standardised screening tool such as AMT (abbreviated mental test) or MMSE (mini-mental state examination), including tests for attention (e.g. serial 7s, WORLD backwards).
- Asterixis can be seen in hepatic encephalopathy.
- Tremors can be seen in alcohol withdrawal and delirium tremens.
- Check reflexes looking for clonus as can be seen in serotonin syndrome or hyperthyroidism.

Assessment tools in the ICU

Several methods have been developed and validated especially to diagnose delirium in ICU patients, but the Confusion Assessment Method for the Intensive Care Unit (CAM–ICU) and the Intensive Care Delirium Screening Checklist (ICDSC) are the most frequently employed tools for this purpose. The CAM-ICU and the ICDSC are good screening tools for delirium in ICU patients, and the CAM-ICU is an excellent diagnostic tool for delirium in critically ill ICU patients.

The Confusion Assessment Method for the Intensive Care Unit (CAM–ICU)

The CAM–ICU is based on the CAM, reflecting the DSM-III-R[19] criteria, and is designed for patients with limited communication abilities.

This scale contains four features with two levels (absent and present):

1. acute onset and fluctuating course

2. inattention

3. altered level of consciousness

4. disorganised thinking.

Feature 1 scores as absent or present; feature 2 includes 'recognising letters' scores as number of errors (more than two scores as present); feature 3 scores the Richmond Agitation Assessment Scale (RASS) other than alert and calm (RASS = 0) as present; and feature 4 includes simple questions and instructions, with a combined number of errors of more than one scored as present. Features 1 plus 2 and either 3 or 4 scored as present indicates presence of delirium.

The Intensive Care Delirium Screening Checklist (ICDSC)

The ICDSC is a screening instrument that includes eight items based on DSM-IV-TR[20] criteria specifically designed for the intensive care setting. It has two score points: absent and present. This scale was designed for patients with limited communication abilities, such as intubated patients.

The items include the assessment of:

1. consciousness (comatose, soporose, awake or hypervigilant)

2. orientation

3. hallucinations or delusions

4. psychomotor activity

5. inappropriate speech or mood

6. attentiveness

7. sleep–wake cycle disturbances

8. fluctuation of symptomatology.

The maximum score is 8, and scores of more than 3 indicate the presence of delirium. Each item is rated based on the patient's behaviour over the previous 24 hours.

Bedside tests

Most of the 'bedside tests' involve different types of attention and differ in terms of the demands placed on other cognitive domains. Indeed, deficits in multiple cognitive systems including language, memory, perceptual, motor and executive functions can all contribute to poor neuropsychological test performance.

Investigations

The investigations listed in Box 2.3 are almost always indicated in patients with delirium in order to identify the underlying cause:

BOX 2.3 INVESTIGATIONS

- Full blood count including C-reactive protein (CRP)
- Urea and electrolytes, calcium
- Liver function tests
- Glucose
- Chest X-ray
- Electrocardiography
- Blood cultures
- Pulse oximetry
- Urinalysis

Other investigations may be indicated according to the findings from the history and examination (see Box 2.4).

BOX 2.4 FURTHER INVESTIGATIONS

- Computed tomography (CT) of the head
- Electroencephalogram (EEG)
- Thyroid function tests
- B_{12} and folate
- Arterial blood gases
- Specific cultures, e.g. urine, sputum
- Lumbar puncture

Brain neuroimaging

The aim of brain neuroimaging is to identify stroke, haemorrhage or trauma as causes of delirium. The diagnostic yield of computed tomography (CT) in determining the cause of delirium is low, but may be indicated in some high-risk patients. For patients with pre-existing cognitive impairment who have other identified conditions that can precipitate delirium, such as dehydration or infection, brain imaging is unlikely to change management.

Observational, mostly retrospective, studies identified abnormal brain imaging in CT scans in people aged over 70 years presenting with acute confusion and:

- new focal neurological signs (defined as acute onset dysphasia, visual field defect, pyramidal or cerebellar signs)

- presenting after a fall

- a reduced level of consciousness (Glasgow Coma Score <9)

- a head injury (in patients of any age) *or*

- taking anticoagulant therapy.

Cerebral atrophy is more likely in patients presenting with delirium than without. This in itself, however, is *not* a useful finding in making a diagnosis of delirium or changing medical management.

Although studying how structural lesions affect phenotype has been insightful in other diagnoses, relevant structural abnormalities are usually absent in delirium. Understanding which regions are functionally dynamically affected in delirium, such as a 'default mode network', may implicate cerebral pathways and highlight novel biomarkers and therapeutic targets.

Although many patients with delirium have an underlying dementia or structural brain lesion (e.g. previous stroke), CT has been shown to be unhelpful if used on a routine basis to identify a cause for delirium, and could be reserved for those patients in whom an intracranial lesion is suspected.[21]

Indications for the use of CT scanning include:

- focal neurological signs

- confusion developing after head injury

- confusion developing after a fall

- evidence of raised intracranial pressure.

Other modalities of neuroimaging in delirium include MRI, fMRI and NIRS.

Electroencephalogram (EEG)

Delirium is associated with slowing of EEG background activity, specifically an increased relative delta power at 1–4Hz. EEG-based monitoring and quantification could have great potential for predicting and detecting delirium in routine daily practice, as it is objective and applicable in all patients despite language or sensory barriers.

EEG may be useful where there is difficulty in the following situations:

- differentiating delirium from dementia
- differentiating delirium from non-convulsive status epilepticus and temporal lobe epilepsy
- identifying those patients in whom the delirium is due to a focal intracranial lesion, rather than a global abnormality.

There are problems. Spatial resolution is poor, hampering anatomical interferences. Artefacts can be a problem. The complex signal can be prone to misinterpretation.

Currently, EEG is not performed routinely in patients with delirium, but it could be considered when there is a suspicion of epileptic activity or non-convulsive status epilepticus as a cause of a patient's delirium.

'Deep learning' algorithms can learn task-relevant features from raw signals, reducing the need to handcraft features or biomarkers for a specific task. This ability is promising for EEG-based tracking of level of consciousness and delirium, where human experts may not be able to identify all features in EEG waveforms relevant to the brain states of interest.[22]

In future, EEG might be able to be used to predict which patients might benefit best from neuropharmacological interventions.

Lumbar puncture

Although various abnormalities have been seen in the cerebrospinal fluid of patients with delirium, routine lumbar puncture is not helpful in identifying an underlying cause for the delirium. It should therefore be reserved for those in whom there is reason to suspect a cause such as meningitis. This might include patients with the following features: meningism, headache and fever.

Lumbar puncture is not a straightforward procedure and such an invasive investigation may be totally impractical or cause further distress to someone who may be confused or agitated. There is also a risk of adverse events, such as infection, causing spinal haematoma, cerebrospinal fluid (CSF) leak or low-pressure CSF headache.

Potential impact of diagnostic errors

It is possible that physicians of patients with delirium often incorrectly turn to past psychiatric diagnoses and/or are distracted by the presence of pain and, thus, fail to accurately diagnose delirium.[23]

In a different study, of 221 consultations over a five-year period, 46% were misdiagnosed by the house staff. House staff on the general medicine wards and the non-ICU environment did significantly better than those on the surgical wards and intensive care units.[24]

It has long been suggested that the hypoactive form of delirium is frequently misdiagnosed as depression, which underscores the importance of considering delirium in the differential diagnosis of patients' mood disturbance. Its presence is frequently not recognised and management remains suboptimal.

Endnotes

1   Fong, T.G., Tulebaev, S.R. and Inouye, S.K. (2009) 'Delirium in elderly adults: Diagnosis, prevention and treatment.' *Nature Reviews Neurology 5*, 210–220. Accessed on 29/11/2019 at www.ncbi.nlm.nih.gov/pmc/articles/PMC3065676.

2   Inouye, S.K., van Dyck, C.H., Alessi, C.A., Balkin, S., Siegal, A.P. and Horwitz, R.I. (1990) 'Clarifying confusion: The Confusion Assessment Method. A new method for detection of delirium.' *Annals of Internal Medicine 113*, 12, 941–948. Accessed on 29/11/2019 at www.ncbi.nlm.nih.gov/pubmed/2240918.

3   Wei, L.A., Fearing, M.A., Sternberg, E.J. and Inouye, S.K. (2008) 'The Confusion Assessment Method: A systematic review of current usage.' *Journal of the American Geriatrics Society 56*, 5, 823–830. Accessed on 29/11/2019 at www.ncbi.nlm.nih.gov/pubmed/18384586.

4   Inouye, S.K. (2014) *The CAM-S Training Manual and Coding Guide*. Boston, MA: Hospital Elder Life Program. Accessed on 16/12/2019 at http://www.hospitalelderlifeprogram.org/uploads/disclaimers/CAM-S_Training_Manual.pdf.

5   Marcantonio, E.R., Ngo, L.H., O'Connor, M., Jones, R.N. *et al.* (2014) '3D-CAM: Derivation and validation of a 3-minute diagnostic interview for CAM-defined delirium. A cross-sectional diagnostic test study.' *Annals of Internal Medicine 161*, 8, 554–561. Accessed on 29/11/2019 at www.ncbi.nlm.nih.gov/pubmed/25329203.

6   Steis, M.R., Evans, L., Hirschmann, K.B., Hanlon, A. *et al.* (2012) 'Screening for delirium using family caregivers: Convergent validity of the Family Confusion Assessment Method and interviewer-rated Confusion Assessment Method.' *Journal of the American Geriatrics Society 60*, 11, 2121–2126. Accessed on 29/11/2019 at www.ncbi.nlm.nih.gov/pubmed/23039310.

7   Shenkin, S.D., Fox, C., Godfrey, M., Siddiqi, N. *et al.* (2019) 'Delirium detection in older acute medical inpatients: A multicentre prospective comparative diagnostic tests accuracy study of the 4AT and the confusion assessment method.' *BMC Medicine 17*, 138. Accessed on 28/11/2019 at https://bmcmedicine.biomedcentral.com/articles/10.1186/s12916-019-1367-9.

8   Health Improvement Scotland (2019) *SIGN 157: Risk Reduction and Management of Delirium. A National Clinical Guideline*. Accessed on 28/11/2019 at www.sign.ac.uk/assets/sign157.pdf.

9   World Health Organization (1992) *The ICD-10 Classification of Mental and Behavioural Disorders: Clinical Descriptions and Diagnostic Guidelines*. Geneva: WHO.

10   American Psychiatric Association (2013) *Diagnostic and Statistical Manual of Mental Disorders, Fifth Edition (DSM-5)*. Washington, DC: APA.

11   Lucke, J.A., de Gelder, J., Blomaard, L.C., Heringhaus, C. *et al.* (2019) 'Vital signs and impaired cognition in older emergency department patients: The APOP study.' *PLOS One 14*, 6, e02185596. Accessed on 29/11/2019 at https://journals.plos.org/plosone/article?id=10.1371/journal.pone.0218596.

12   Ellis, G. and Sevdalis, N. (2019) 'Understanding and improving multidisciplinary team working in geriatric medicine.' *Age and Ageing 48*, 4, 498–505. Accessed on 29/11/2019 at https://academic.oup.com/ageing/article/48/4/498/5374432.

13   Johnson, M.H. (2001) 'Assessing confused patients.' *Journal of Neurology, Neurosurgery and Psychiatry 71*, i7–i12. Accessed on 29/11/2019 at https://jnnp.bmj.com/content/71/suppl_1/i7.

14   Meagher, D.J. and Trzpacz, P.T. (2000) 'Motoric subtypes of delirium.' *Seminars in Clinical Neuropsychiatry 5*, 2, 75–85. Accessed on 29/11/2019 at www.ncbi.nlm.nih.gov/pubmed/10837096.

15 Think delirium: https://learn.nes.nhs.scot/2442/rrheal/education-networks/rgh-education-network/think-delirium-improving-the-care-for-older-people-delirium-toolkit.

16 Williams, B. (2019) 'The National Early Warning Score and the acutely confused patient.' *Clinical Medicine 19*, 2, 190–191. Accessed on 16/12/2019 at www.ncbi.nlm.nih.gov/pmc/articles/PMC6454357.

17 See www.bapen.org.uk/pdfs/must/must-full.pdf.

18 See www.drugbank.ca/drugs/DB03575.

19 American Psychiatric Association (1987) *Diagnostic and Statistical Manual of Mental Disorders, Third Edition Revised (DSM-III-R)*. Washington, DC: APA.

20 American Psychiatric Association (1994) *Diagnostic and Statistical Manual of Mental Disorders, Fourth Edition, Text Revision (DMS-IV-TR)*. Washington, DC: APA.

21 Khoo, S.B. (2011) 'Acute grief with delirium in an elderly: Holistic care.' *Malaysian Family Physician 6*, 2–3, 51–57. Accessed on 29/11/2019 at www.ncbi.nlm.nih.gov/pmc/articles/PMC4170417.

22 Sun, H., Kimchi, E., Akeju, O., Nagaraj. S.B. *et al.* (2019) 'Automated tracking of level of consciousness and delirium in critical illness using deep learning.' *NPJ Digital Medicine 2*, 89. Accessed on 29/11/2019 at www.ncbi.nlm.nih.gov/pmc/articles/PMC6733797.

23 Kishi, Y., Kato, M., Okuyama, T., Hosaka, T. *et al.* (2007) 'Delirium: Patient characteristics that predict a missed diagnosis at psychiatric consultation.' *General Hospital Psychiatry 29*, 5, 442–445. Accessed on 29/11/2019 at www.ncbi.nlm.nih.gov/pubmed/17888812.

24 Armstrong, S.C., Cozza, K.L. and Watanabe, K.S. (1997) 'The misdiagnosis of delirium.' *Psychosomatics 38*, 5, 433–439. Accessed on 29/11/2019 at www.ncbi.nlm.nih.gov/pubmed/9314712.

3

Delirium risk reduction and prevention

LEARNING OBJECTIVES

In an ideal world, all delirium would and could be prevented. It has become realistic to think about reducing the risk of delirium, knowing that particular types of patients might be especially susceptible. This has led to a variety of different approaches, ranging from individual motivational change to systems behavioural change.

'Prevention is better than cure'

Evidence for delirium prevention has been incorporated into national guidelines in Australia, the United Kingdom and the United States, and yet direct patient-care activities such as assessment, family/patient interaction, nutrition and mobility required in delirium prevention are not prioritised and are sometimes missed out or left partially completed.[1]

It is estimated that about 30% of delirium is preventable.[2] It is generally accepted that prevention is better than cure. This adage is particularly pertinent to delirium. Various pharmacological and non-pharmacological approaches to treatment of established delirium have been tested, yet a 'cure' for delirium has proven elusive.

Primary prevention of delirium is therefore of critical importance and practical significance to patients, families and healthcare institutions because of the physical, emotional and financial burdens of caring for the older adult who is suffering from delirium.

Many of the acute factors triggering delirium or lowering the threshold of risk are modifiable. Studies of patients in hospital have shown that it can be beneficial to use care plans that target the main risk factors for delirium – for example, providing better lighting and signs to avoid disorientation, avoiding unnecessary use of catheters to help prevent infection, avoiding medications that increase delirium risk.[3]

Delirium may even persist far beyond the hospital stay, with documented episodes lasting weeks to months. Delirium prevention therefore must be communicated across the community in all care settings. Between 3% and 16% of patients are estimated to be discharged from hospitals with delirium.[4] Delirium at discharge may be on the rise due to the under-recognition of delirium symptoms and the pressure to shorten the length of hospital stays. (A brief account of the plethora of outcomes after an episode of delirium is given in Chapter 8.)

How to tackle delirium prevention has been the focus of a large body of professional-quality improvement work in many care settings. To be feasible and acceptable, a 'delirium prevention programme' needs 'buy in', both at the administrative level and by people providing care. It is important that all stakeholders find ownership in the intervention. Stakeholders must be willing to change their practice to conform to what the delirium prevention programme requires. This itself requires effective clinical leadership. Quality improvement is described in detail in Chapter 12. In recent years, the role of educational intervention has also been assessed in relation to prevention. The efficacy of educational initiatives is likely to result from enhancing awareness of delirium risk factors and the identification of 'at-risk' patients (see Chapter 13).

Data indicating that delirium can be successfully prevented through the active targeting of modifiable risk factors are not new. Methodological difficulties and inconsistencies have affected the generalisation of results and the clear establishment of protocols and strategies.

The **MRC framework for evaluating complex interventions**[5] has been used to design an intervention to prevent delirium in care homes (entitled 'Stop Delirium!') and demonstrated its feasibility.[6] Stop Delirium! is an enhanced educational package, incorporating additional strategies to change practice, designed to support staff to target common risk factors for delirium in residents.

Sources of health promotion

While guidelines are useful, guidelines alone are insufficient to effect change in practice and service delivery in this area. Knowledge within organisations is both codified and non-codified. There has been an impressive increase in the amount and availability of health promotion information, both reliable and unreliable.

Family might still be ranked ahead of health books, newspapers, television news, magazines with regard to reliability.[7] This may be related in part to the relative importance of family members in the social networks of persons experiencing illness.

There are currently no charities specifically related to delirium offering free information, although delirium is a subject of interest to dementia charities.[8]

Motivational factors

Motivation is a complex neuroscientific construct, elegant syntheses of which exist elsewhere.[9]

It encompasses a variety of processes, including a drive to homeostasis, as well as the use of appetite- and aversive-reward-driven mechanisms to control action and to guide behaviour.

Motivation may be internally or externally driven.

Encouraging behavioural change has been an area of intense scrutiny for some time. It is popular to contrast 'carrots' with 'sticks'. Some use some form of incentive to reward individuals for adopting behaviours that protect against disease and promote health; others take a more punitive approach to 'put people off' certain behaviours.[10]

There are various examples of models of motivational change.

Two examples are:

1. The **transtheoretical model** is an integrative, biopsychosocial model to conceptualise the process of intentional behaviour change.

2. **Festinger's cognitive dissonance theory** describes how, when there is a discrepancy between two beliefs or between a belief and an action, a person will act to resolve conflict.

Delirium prevention

Engaging in preventative action requires knowledge at different levels: about risk factors that may predispose a patient to a specific issue, and about the kinds of interventions or practices that have the potential to be a meaningful intervention in reducing the modifiable risk. It also requires reliable systems to identify those at risk, and the recruitment of staff to carry out practices which contribute to risk reduction.

Delirium prediction and electronic patient records

'Delirium prediction rules' contain independent risk factors for delirium that are combined together into a computational algorithm; the delirium prediction rule is then validated in a separate population. A dynamic model can be critical for accurate real-time risk estimation, because some risk factors may have only short-term implications for risk or may emerge during the hospitalisation itself.

In 2010, the National Institute for Clinical and Healthcare Excellence (NICE) published a systematic review and meta-analysis of the best available evidence for delirium risk factors. The meta-analysis identified six independent risk factors for delirium to produce a NICE 'delirium prediction tool':[11] impaired baseline cognition, vision impairment, severity of illness, fracture, infection and age.

Adoption of electronic medical records in hospitals generates a large amount of data, not all of which feels completely relevant. Healthcare professionals can easily lose sight of the important qualitative insights of patients' clinical and medical history. Machine learning algorithms, although only recently developed, have already proved their significance in healthcare research and many other fields of medicine. They might yet be useful in delirium prediction. Algorithms, however, are not infallible and may be subject to biases. The biases include those related to missing data and patients not identified by algorithms, sample size and underestimation, and misclassification and measurement error.[12]

Risk factor assessment

When people first present to hospital or long-term care, they should be assessed for the following risk factors. If any of these risk factors is present, it could be argued that the person is *at risk of delirium*:

- older people

- older people on multiple medicines

- cognitive impairment or central neurology

- current hip fracture

- visual or hearing impairment

- severe illness (a clinical condition that is deteriorating or is at risk of deterioration).

Introduction to prediction models

Although research to date has failed to identify a clear unifying pathology for delirium, there is a body of work looking to define **risk algorithms** to identify patients at risk, and ultimately to intervene and prevent delirium from occurring in the first place.

Prediction models allow clinicians to forecast which individuals are at a higher risk for the development of a particular disease, and target specific interventions at the identified risk profile. Such models may aid clinical decision-making and establishing priorities regarding the use of 'delirium preventative measures'. They are intended to improve patients' outcomes across specific care settings.

A **'severity model'** would identify patients who are likely to become afflicted by the severest delirium, and therefore are most likely to benefit from a delirium prevention plan.[13]

Delirium presents a number of context-specific problems. For example, the risk factors of delirium in ICU patients are different among studies but might include age and exposure to sedatives and analgesics.

Widening preventative care also enables family members to be more fully informed about a patient's risk of developing delirium and to be actively involved in someone's care. An important context is that involvement of family in patient care in the ICU is stimulated by many ICU societies worldwide, and might even increase the prevalence of interventions for delirium prevention and treatment in the ICU.

PRE-DELIRIC

The PRE-DELIRIC model has been internationally validated, although its true predictive value can vary from one ICU to another.

The PRE-DELIRIC model was created in 2013 in the Netherlands based on a systemic review of delirium risk factors.[14] The model includes ten objectively and clearly defined risk factors known within 24 hours of admission to the ICU.[15]

The Inouye and Charpentier prediction model for delirium

In 1996, Inouye and Charpentier developed and validated a prediction model for delirium based on precipitating factors during hospitalisation.[16]

A simple prediction model based on the presence of five precipitating factors can be used to identify elderly medical patients at high risk for delirium.

Five independent precipitating factors for delirium were identified:

1. use of physical restraints

2. malnutrition

3. more than three medications

4. use of bladder catheter

5. any iatrogenic event.

Each precipitating factor preceded the onset of delirium by more than 24 hours.

The general approach to multicomponent interventions

Multicomponent interventions are a fairly heterogeneous group of measures that typically target multiple delirium risk factors in a systematic manner.

The following components could be considered as part of a package of care for patients at risk of developing delirium:

- orientation

- early mobilisation

- pain control

- prevention, early identification and treatment of post-operative complications

- maintaining optimal hydration and nutrition

- regulation of bladder and bowel function

- provision of oxygen, if required.

Environmental factors such as sleep disturbance and emotional distress may also prevent delirium from resolving in the hospital. Therefore, one approach (called 'multicomponent interventions') to preventing delirium is to target these multiple risk factors. Improvements, such as reduced duration of delirium, have been claimed, but the benefits in the real-world setting are modest.

The most robust evidence for delirium prevention relates to *non-pharmacological* multicomponent interventions involving assessment of patients to identify and then modify risk factors associated with delirium. Although evidence and consensus support the application of multicomponent strategies in delirium prevention, efforts to apply the trial design to real life have been beset by heterogeneity and inconsistency in the nature of the interventions.

All too often pharmacological management has been adopted in the clinical setting over a holistic approach. However, as well as improvement in patient outcomes, multicomponent delirium prevention strategies have resulted in significant cost savings to healthcare providers. It is clear therefore that delirium prevention strategies are crucial to reduce the health burden and economic consequences of delirium.

A recent Cochrane review looked at 'Interventions to prevent delirium in hospitalised patients'.[17] The authors reviewed the evidence for the effectiveness of interventions for preventing delirium in hospitalised patients, not including those on intensive care units (ICUs) (specialised wards for the care of critically ill patients).

Introduction to HELP
Various interventions have been tested across a number of jurisdictions, in different health systems, in diverse settings (medical, surgical and intensive care units) and employ varied modes of delivery.

Prof. Sharon Inouye, a professor at Harvard, has led globally in identifying the precipitating factors of delirium and implementing coherent, intelligent and humanistic strategies to prevent it in older patients admitted to hospital. Service models include the **Hospital Elder Life Program** (HELP), which uses a skilled interdisciplinary team assisted by trained volunteers and proactive geriatric consultation with targeted recommendations based on a structured protocol.

HELP involves the implementation of practical tailored interventions to prevent delirium, targeting reorientation, early mobilisation, therapeutic activities, hydration, nutrition, sleep strategies and hearing and visual adaptations, by trained volunteers.

The HELP program's website has a list of ten tips for friends and family of older patients, the population most vulnerable to developing delirium during a hospitalisation.[18]

The Fam-HELP program
Family carers can be defined as a spouse, adult child, other relative, partner or friend who has a personal relationship with and provides a broad range of unpaid assistance for another.

Prevention and management strategies can involve the older person's family in assisting the older person to move regularly, to eat and drink well, to remain independent in activities of living and social interaction, and to use their visual and hearing aids when required.

The protocols of the Fam-HELP program are considered to be amenable to family implementation.

The ABCDE bundle

Current non-pharmacological interventions involve risk factor identification, with situation-specific modification, and implementation of evidence-based practices, when clinically appropriate, such as awakening and breathing, coordination with target-based sedation, delirium monitoring, and exercise/ early mobility ('ABCDE Bundle'). This intervention is considered in much more detail in Chapter 7.

Pharmacological approaches in prevention of delirium

Delirium pharmacological treatment studies are hard to do, for a number of reasons:[19]

- For delirium treatment (as opposed to prevention), you must identify and enrol individuals with delirium; this requires active surveillance on the part of the investigator.

- Delirious patients often lack capacity, and obtaining consent from a substitute decision-maker may be challenging.

- These are sick, vulnerable patients, and developing a standardised treatment protocol that fits all of them is difficult.

- Identifying the appropriate outcomes is challenging; for prevention, the key outcome is delirium, but for delirium treatment, the key outcomes are less clear.

Many pharmacological strategies have been investigated to prevent delirium, although the data have been inconsistent and conflicting.

Analgosedation is defined as either analgesia-first sedation or analgesia-based sedation.[20] The primary focus of this regimen is to make the treatment of pain a priority in providing sedatives, aiming to achieve and maintain a mild level of sedation. Analgosedation that spares opioid and sedative use has potential advantages in preventing delirium.

Steroid administration during critical illness has been associated with transition to delirium.

Attentional disturbances are caused by dysfunction in the ascending reticular activating system, which regulates arousal. Arousal is controlled by multiple neurotransmitters released from neurons in the ascending reticular activating system and brainstem. Noradrenaline is especially implicated here.

Dopamine is a neurotransmitter, and medications that potentiate its effects can cause psychosis whereas those that block its effects are used as antipsychotics. Medications with anticholinergic properties can precipitate delirium, potentially through altered neurotransmission or altered neuro-inflammation.

Gamma-aminobutyric acid is the primary inhibitory neurotransmitter. It plays a principal role in reducing neuronal excitability throughout the nervous system, thereby preventing overstimulation and stress reactions.

Reserve

Brain reserve is conceptualised as a passive process deriving from the brain structure – in particular, morphological attributes of the cerebral cortex – but cognitive reserve refers to the brain actively coping with an insult.[21] Studies have elucidated vulnerability factors for delirium including factors such as frailty, cognitive impairment, vision or hearing impairment, and comorbidity. Cognitive and brain reserve concepts represent important new ways of framing a vulnerability to delirium.[22]

Cognitive impairment is probably more common among patients presenting for surgery than is generally assumed. These factors contribute to individual brain and cognitive reserve, which might provide protection from short- and long-term cognitive changes, including dementia.

Avoiding post-operative cognitive dysfunction

Post-operative cognitive dysfunction remains a poorly understood and highly variable neuropsychiatric syndrome characterised by neurocognitive dysfunction, which frequently manifests in the hours or days following surgery. Proper classification of the condition remains problematic and may encompass a spectrum of acute confusional states and low-grade encephalopathic states.[23]

There are a number of important pre-operative factors that increase the risk of developing delirium after surgery, including advancing age, cognitive and functional impairment, alcohol abuse, depression, increasing duration of anaesthesia, post-operative complications and abnormal pre-operative electrolytes.

Several hospital-related precipitating factors also exist, including physical restraints, malnutrition and dehydration, urinary catheters, three or more new medications, and any iatrogenic event.[24]

Many of these factors are not modifiable.

On a practical note, using monitoring to avoid episodes of deep anaesthesia in patients aged over 60 under general anaesthesia for surgery lasting more than one hour can significantly reduce the risk of developing post-operative delirium.

Endnotes

1   Grealish, L., Todd, J.A., Krug, M. and Teodorczuk, A. (2019) 'Education for delirium prevention: Knowing, meaning and doing.' *Nurse Education in Practice 40*, 102622. Accessed on 29/11/2019 at www.ncbi.nlm.nih.gov/pubmed/31521042.

2   Fong, T.G., Tulebaev, S.R. and Inouye, S.K. (2009) 'Delirium in elderly adults: Diagnosis, prevention and treatment.' *Nature Reviews Neurology 5*, 210–220. Accessed on 29/11/2019 at www.ncbi.nlm.nih.gov/pmc/articles/PMC3065676.

3   Clegg, A., Siddiqi, N., Heaven, A., Young, J. and Holt, R. (2014) 'Interventions for preventing delirium in older people in institutional long-term care.' *Cochrane Database of Systematic Reviews 31*, 1, CD009537. Accessed on 29/11/2019 at www.ncbi.nlm.nih.gov/pubmed/24488526.

4   Kosar, C.M., Thomas, K.S., Inouye, S.K. and Mor, V. (2017) 'Delirium during postacute nursing home admission and risk for adverse outcomes.' *Journal of the American Geriatrics Society 65*, 7, 1470–1475. Accessed on 29/11/2019 at www.ncbi.nlm.nih.gov/pmc/articles/PMC5515080.

5   See https://mrc.ukri.org/documents/pdf/complex-interventions-guidance.

6   Siddiqi, N., Young, J., Cheater, F.M. and Harding, R.A. (2008) 'Educating staff working in long-term care about delirium: The Trojan horse for improving quality of care?' *Journal of Psychosomatic Research 65*, 3, 261–266. Accessed on 29/11/2019 at www.ncbi.nlm.nih.gov/pubmed/18707949.

7   MacHaffie, S. (2002) 'Health promotion information: Sources and significance for those with serious and persistent mental illness.' *Archives of Psychiatric Nursing 16*, 6, 263–274. Accessed on 29/11/2019 at www.ncbi.nlm.nih.gov/pubmed/12567374.

8   See e.g. www.alzheimers.org.uk/get-support/daily-living/delirium.

9   Berridge, K.C. (2004) 'Motivation concepts in behavioural neuroscience.' *Physiology and Behavior 81*, 179–209. Accessed on 29/11/2019 at https://lsa.umich.edu/psych/research&labs/berridge/publications/Berridge%20Motivation%20concepts%20Physio%20&%20Beh%202004.pdf.

10   Blacksher, E. (2008) 'Carrots and sticks to promote healthy behaviors: A policy update.' *Hastings Center Report 38*, 3, 13–16. Accessed on 29/11/2019 at www.ncbi.nlm.nih.gov/pubmed/18581931.

11   Kostas, T.R.M., Zimmerman, K.M. and Rudolph, J.L. (2013) 'Improving delirium care: Prevention, monitoring, and assessment.' *Neurohospitalist 3*, 4, 194–202. Accessed on 29/11/2019 at www.ncbi.nlm.nih.gov/pmc/articles/PMC3810833.

12   Gianfrancesco, M.A., Tamang, S., Yazdany, J. and Schmajuk, G. (2018) 'Potential biases in machine learning algorithms using electronic health record data.' *JAMA Internal Medicine 178*, 11, 1544–1547. Accessed on 29/11/2019 at www.ncbi.nlm.nih.gov/pubmed/30128552.

13   Lindroth, H., Bratzke, L., Twadell, S., Rowley, P. *et al.* (2018) 'Derivation of a simple postoperative delirium incidence and severity prediction model.' *bioRxiv.* Accessed on 29/11/2019 at www.biorxiv.org/content/10.1101/426148v1.

14   Linkaitė, G., Riaukam M., Bunevičiūtė, I. and Vosylius, S. (2018) 'Evaluation of PRE-DELIRIC (PREdiction of DELIRium in ICu patients) delirium prediction model for the patients in the intensive care unit.' *Acta Medica Lituanica 25*, 1, 14–22. Accessed on 29/11/2019 at www.ncbi.nlm.nih.gov/pmc/articles/PMC6008005.

15   These ten factors are: age, Acute Physiology and Chronic Health Evaluation II (APACHE II) score, coma, urgent admission (unplanned ICU admission), admission category (surgical, medical, trauma, neurology/neurosurgical), infection, use of sedatives, morphine use (three dosage groups), serum urea and metabolic acidosis.

16   Inouye, S.K. and Charpentier, P.A. (1996) 'Precipitating factors for delirium in hospitalized elderly persons. Predictive model and interrelationship with baseline vulnerability.' *JAMA 275*, 11, 852–857. Accessed 17/02/2020 at https://www.ncbi.nlm.nih.gov/pubmed/8596223.

17   Siddiqi, N., Harrison, J.K., Clegg, A., Teale, E.A. *et al.* (2016) 'Interventions to prevent delirium in hospitalised patients, not including those on intensive care units.' Cochrane Library. Accessed on 29/11/2019 at www.cochrane.org/CD005563/DEMENTIA_interventions-prevent-delirium-hospitalised-patients-not-including-those-intensive-care-units.

18   Hospital Elder Life Program (2019) 'What you can do if your family member is delirious.' Accessed on 29/11/2019 at www.hospitalelderlifeprogram.org/for-family-members/what-you-can-do.

19   Marcantonio, E.R. (2019) 'Old habits die hard: Antipsychotics for treatment of delirium.' *Annals of Internal Medicine 171*, 7, 516–517. Accessed on 29/11/2019 at https://annals.org/aim/fullarticle/2749505/old-habits-die-hard-antipsychotics-treatment-delirium.

20   Devlin, J.W., Skrobik, Y., Gélinas, C., Needham, D.M. *et al.* (2018) 'Executive summary: Clinical practice guidelines for the prevention and management of pain, agitation/sedation, delirium, immobility, and sleep disruption in adult patients in the ICU.' *Critical Care Medicine 46*, 9, 1532–1548. Accessed on 29/11/2019 at www.ncbi.nlm.nih.gov/pubmed/30113371.

21   Stern, Y. (2009) 'Cognitive reserve.' *Neuropsychologica 47*, 10, 2015–2028. Accessed on 29/11/2019 at www.ncbi.nlm.nih.gov/pmc/articles/PMC2739591.

22   Jones, R.N., Fong, T.G., Metzger, E., Tulebaev, S. *et al.* (2010) 'Aging, brain disease, and reserve: Implications for delirium.' *American Journal of Geriatric Psychiatry 18*, 2, 117–127. Accessed on 15/01/2020 at www.ncbi.nlm.nih.gov/pmc/articles/PMC2848522.

23   El-Gabalawy, R., Patel, R., Kilborn, K., Blaney, C. *et al.* (2017) 'A Novel Stress-Diathesis Model to Predict Risk of Post-operative Delirium: Implications for Intra-operative Management.' In L. Fernandes and H. Wang (eds) *Mood and Cognition in Old Age.* Frontiers Media. Accessed on 16/12/2019 at https://www.frontiersin.org/articles/10.3389/fnagi.2017.00274/full.

24   Holroyd, J.M., Abelseth, G.A., Khandwala, F., Silvius, J.L. *et al.* (2010) 'A pragmatic study exploring the prevention of delirium among hospitalized older hip fracture patients: Applying evidence to routine clinical practice using clinical decision support.' *Implementation Science.* Accessed on 29/11/2019 at https://implementationscience.biomedcentral.com/articles/10.1186/1748-5908-5-81.

4

Person-centred delirium care

LEARNING OBJECTIVES

It seems intuitive that delirium care should be 'person-centred', but it is an altogether different issue to examine to what extent personhood can and should be respected. It might also be instructive to consider various angles of care, which are centred on the person, carers (friends/family) and relationships.

Introduction

Healthcare professionals should follow established pathways of good care to manage patients with delirium, but the challenge of 'person-centred care' cannot be underestimated.

One massive issue is that the patient with delirium to all intents and purposes is behaving like 'a different person' – making person-centred care challenging.

It would also be churlish to ignore too another 'elephant in the room' – that there are wider 'system factors'. Barriers to implementing person-centred care in delirium can easily be witnessed in a recent article:[1]

> Staff commitment to placing the person at the centre of care was impeded by situational circumstances. The continuous telephone calls, required to coordinate admissions and discharges from the ward, regularly interrupted conversations with patients, families and other staff. The invisibility of the family in the documents suggested an impediment to continuity of care between home, hospital, and home again.

John Locke famously argued that a person is 'a thinking intelligent being, that has reason and reflection, and can consider itself as itself, the same thinking thing in different times and places'.

The focus on 'diagnostic labelling' in acute care contexts, however, potentially fails to take full account of the complex array of social, psychological and cultural factors that shape health and wellbeing, and might inadvertently attract stigma.[2] Patients with delirium have multiple needs that cut across disease categories and require creative, reflective approaches to care, for which protocols are insufficient.

The emotional care and security of patients with cognitive impairment using person-centred care advocated by pioneer Tom Kitwood has consistently been recognised as 'best practice'.

Critical to the integration of delirium detection and management on acute wards should be those working practices that place value on person-centred approaches. It can be difficult not to allow 'diagnostic labelling' trump respect for personhood in carefully streamed care pathways.

In 2019 Rahman noted on the blog of the British Geriatrics Society:[3]

> An alternative approach could be that we have more holistic person-centred geriatrics wards, where people are not streamed by diagnoses. This might be advisable, not least because diagnoses overlap commonly in geriatrics, and with the benefit of hindsight, may turn out to be incorrect.

Neurologically, the 'self' is clearly a multidimensional construct, composed of multiple functionally independent systems, including episodic memory, semantic memory and autobiographical memory.[4] This might be of some relevance to delirium.

Challenging stereotypes

Stereotypes are unchallenged myths or overstated beliefs associated with a category which are widespread and entrenched in verbal, written and visual contexts within society.

Stereotypes of ageing include assumptions and generalisations about how people at or over a certain age should behave, and what they are likely to experience, without regard for individual differences or unique circumstances. Stereotypes of ageing in contemporary Western culture are primarily negative, depicting later life as a time of ill health, decline, loneliness, dependency, disability and poor physical and mental functioning.

Stereotypes of a person experiencing delirium are relatively under-explored. But a popular depiction is of such a person as 'totally mad'.

At a fundamental level, however, the word '**person**' captures those attributes that represent our humanity and 'constructions'. **Constructions** such as how we, as individuals, think about moral values constituting an identity, how we express political, spiritual or religious beliefs, how we engage emotionally in our social relationships, and the sort of life we want to live are all framed through attributes as persons. For example, research has consistently linked indices of religious coping to measures of health and wellbeing, a major source of support and hope, among diverse groups recovering from physical and mental illness or facing critical life events. Religiosity in delirium may even affect mortality.[5]

Culture change

It is hoped[6] that wider **culture change** in delirium has benefited from seminal work identifying gaps between desired and actual practice, although there is more to achieve. Emerging themes around lack of actual clinical ownership of delirium patients, assumptions that a degree of cognitive impairment is 'normal' in older people and under-appreciation of the phenomenon of distress have led, rightly, to a drive to find and develop more effective educational interventions (Chapter 13). The wider culture of the hospital is a vital indicator of delirium care.

The relative neglect of patients experiencing delirium, whose treatment is both time-consuming and lacking in prestige, may be perpetuated within these hierarchical systems.[7] As an example of where reorienting culture might improve care, it has been noted that delirium recognition might be improved by an ethos of learning and collaboration within an acute admissions unit;[8] a similar approach of embedding a specialist delirium or geriatric medicine team within the acute admissions unit could have a similar positive impact in clinical practice. However, failure rates among organisational change efforts remain frustratingly high, and common obstacles that organisations face in achieving change include failure to sustain the effort over the long term, competing priorities and under-resourcing.[9]

And yet the ultimate goal in improving the quality of person-centred care is highly desirable. 'Culture change' has the potential to improve person-centred care and quality of life for residents, while also improving working conditions for staff.[10] Efforts also often underscore the value of an individual as a unique person with his or her own history, values, ideas and experiences that have shaped who they are. This is even a regulatory goal of the CQC (regulation 9, person-centred care[11]). Recognising and supporting personhood is often found in the context of caring for the person with a cognitive impairment.

Practices that have been described as important for recognising personhood – for instance, life histories – are often not embedded within the routine working practices of an organisation, although exceptions exist. Establishing an amicable relationship involves the development of an amicable and trusting collaboration, whereby all parties recognise the individuality of the other beyond immediate caregiving activities. This might occur by volunteering information, sharing stories and keeping track of events in each other's lives.

The importance of person-centred delirium care

Professors John Young and Sharon Inouye comment:[12]

> Few ill health situations are more degrading to people of any age than loss of reasoning, faculties, and personhood.

Person-centred care has been identified as the ideal approach to caring for people with cognitive impairment, but how this is applied to delirium seems surprisingly under-developed, under-researched and under-implemented. Nonetheless, interviews with carers and others have consistently revealed a shared belief in the importance of **valuing the patient with delirium as a person**, in order to enable a positive caring environment experience. Clinicians tend to emphasise the need for teamwork due to time restraints and the need to manage their competing commitments, alongside the unpredictable nature of caring for a patient with delirium. A lack of time is also often cited by the nurses as one of the main reasons for increased stress and distress when caring for a patient with delirium.

The qualitative research into exploring carers' perceptions of acute hospital care for people with dementia suggest that their experiences are variable.

Compassion is a complex construct that has been defined as 'a deep feeling of connectedness with the experience of human suffering that requires personal knowing of the suffering of others [and] evokes a moral response to the recognised suffering that results in caring that brings comfort to the sufferer'[13] and an ability to relate to the vulnerability of others in meaningful ways. Compassionate care could be the driving force for all clinicians who work in the healthcare field and represents a core value within their professional role. However, our modern-day healthcare culture has progressed to a position where healthcare professionals can feel a need to detach themselves from the emotions of their patients, rather than embed compassion into their daily practice. In caring roles, it is not uncommon for carers to detach themselves emotionally from a person whom they feel they are 'losing'.

What is person-centred delirium care and its relationship to 'personhood'?

An overly biomedical model can easily be criticised because it does not acknowledge 'personhood', in other words contextualise a person within a social construct (such as relationships with others). But it is possibly much worse than that, as delirium is a more drastic manifestation of cognitive changes; at worst, delirium constitutes a temporary 'social death'.[14] Family experiences of absence during an older loved one's delirium, a condition which has an acute onset and which may reverse or persist, have received little consideration to date from this perspective. A 'rebooted' focus on person-centredness in delirium care practice might reflect society's drive to redress the current imbalance in care, moving away from an ethos that is medically dominated, disease-orientated and often fragmented toward one that is relationship-focused, collaborative and holistic.

Person-centredness is generally thought to be based on the promotion of personhood. Thus, at the core of clarifying person-centredness lies a philosophical and theoretical acknowledgement of the nature of personhood. Critically, any act of denying 'personhood' in a patient with delirium is a dangerous, slippery slope. Not only will the delirium in most cases be short-lasting, but also to deny personhood runs the danger of giving licence to care which does not respect dignity or other inalienable human rights. When you fall asleep at night, it is not the case that you no longer exist as a person.

Why is a person-centred, not disease-specific, approach needed?

This is possibly the 'end of the disease era'.[15] There is now increasing awareness of the importance of **multimorbidity**, defined as patients living with two or more chronic health conditions.

Multimorbidity is associated with reduced quality of life, impaired functional status, worse physical and mental health, and increased mortality. The increasing prevalence of multimorbidity, driven by the ageing population, represents a major challenge to all healthcare systems because these patients are heavy users of services. Over half (54%) of older people have at least two chronic conditions, also referred to as multimorbidity.[16] Recommendations based on 'disease-specific guidelines' can be inappropriate for patients with co-existing conditions. Furthermore, segmentation of care by disease means that healthcare for these patients, while potentially very efficient, is often fragmented and poorly coordinated. Patients can sometimes describe wanting one professional to take responsibility for their overall care, and to consider their personal situation and preferences when advising about treatment decisions.

Care of older people with any chronic illness is, rather, often complex, and to deliver person-centred care in this population, a clear understanding of the person's preferences for and goals of care is needed. Person-centred care speaks to providing what is necessary to meet individuals' physical, psychological, social and spiritual needs by focusing on what is important to them. Care preferences can be broadly classified as preferences for the context in which care is delivered; preferences for care relationships; preferences for involvement in care; and preferences for care outcomes, such as comfort versus extending life, or place of death.

Person-centred nursing

Fundamentals of care are integral to ensuring (and teaching) high-quality, compassionate and safe patient care and are essential to nursing.[17] How the fundamentals-of-care framework might be realised in financially constrained, technologically laden health services as our populations become older and sicker is an international priority.[18]

A focus of nursing has tended to be on action rather than outcomes. Nurses were continuously coordinating patient flow, ensuring patients were admitted and discharged efficiently, with limited flexibility around the other care tasks that were required. Routines were inflexible and raised challenges in the care of older people.

A **person-centred nursing framework** was developed by McCormack and McCance in 2010, and was derived from previous empirical research focusing on person-centred practice with older people and the experience of caring in nursing.[19] Person-centredness is an approach to practice established through the formation and development of therapeutic relationships between all care providers, older people and others significant to them in their lives. It is underpinned by values of respect for persons, an individual's right to self-determination, mutual respect and understanding. It is enabled by cultures of empowerment that foster continuous approaches to practice development.

A person-centred framework in nursing might include these constructs:

- Prerequisites focus on the attributes of the people involved.

- The care environment focuses on the context in which care is delivered.

- Person-centred processes focus on delivering care through a range of activities.

- Outcomes, the central component of the framework, are the results of effective person-centred care.

An environment of holistic care

Placing the patient in a central position is essential, concurrent with holistic clinical care. Understanding patients' perceptions provides nurses, physicians and other healthcare workers as well as patients and their family with a better insight into the syndrome. It is likely that nurses who know how patients *perceive* delirium are better equipped to provide more effective person-centred care. When a patient returns to reality, nurses should be able to understand and answer the patient's questions about 'what actually happened'.

Various parties, including patients, family carers and staff, appear to find the admission to hospital of somebody with a cognitive impairment disruptive, and try to respond in ways that help them feel in control in the face of this disruption. The hospital stay can be a particularly stressful and threatening experience for older people with cognitive impairment because of their altered cognitive ability, which affects their capacity to adapt to an unfamiliar setting that entails sharing spaces with strangers, disruption to their daily routines and incursions into their private space.

The global goals in managing a patient with delirium are, arguably, to:

- ensure patient safety

- identify and manage causes, contributors and risk factors

- relieve symptoms.

Long-term care for older people is undergoing significant change internationally. This change reflects a shift in philosophy from an institutional model of care (with an emphasis on illness, disability) to one that truly seeks to celebrate the continuing place of the older person in the community, ensuring the 'person' is at the heart of decision-making about models of care delivery. Moving from patient-centred to person-centred care is an opportunity to break away from any historical association of care of a person experiencing delirium with depersonalised and institutionalised care and revisit the values on which practice might be provided instead.

The goal and overriding challenge of person-centred approaches to care in delirium care is to respect personhood *despite* cognitive impairment. Where the personhood of the individual is recognised and valued, the person with any cognitive impairment is afforded 'standing and status' in society. This approach to the care of the person with any cognitive impairment ideally takes time to develop, and is usually most easily achieved through securing and formulating long-term relationships between any carers and the person experiencing delirium.

Specific aspects of person-centred care

Person-centred delirium care needs to be understood in a broader context than the immediate nurse–patient/family relationship. Despite the existence of expressed person-centred values, care processes often remain routinised and task-focused, with little emphasis on the formation of meaningful relationships.

'Being bored'

A negative consequence of the ward environment can be the experience of boredom, or a lack of occupation. The need for a **'meaningful activity'** programme is often identified by carers, ward staff and patients independently.

Emotions

Although they often have a feeling of happiness at the end of the delirious period, shame and guilt can be present in patients recollecting previous awkward or aggressive behaviour. Patients have an increased risk of developing anxiety disorders following delirium.[20] For example, post-traumatic stress disorder, a severe form of anxiety, is often associated with the post-ICU course.

Sleep and time

Patients might report spontaneously that they notice that the normal day–night circle is disrupted.

Communication

Communication can be very awkward in delirium.

The issue of communication is of vast importance and is considered at length in Chapter 5.

It is felt that when clinicians approach the patient calmly, with understanding and empathy, patients can be reassured. In this way, clinicians can hope that they are not perceived as a 'threat', but rather can prove to be helpful in a difficult situation. The act of listening has an intrinsic therapeutic effect through acknowledging the dignity and personhood of the person speaking.

End-of-life awareness
Issues surrounding end-of-life awareness can evoke significant emotion from carers. Carers might report that their loved one expressed awareness of the dying process or impending death.

Physical symptoms
People might report various physical symptoms, including increased pain, decreased appetite, difficulty breathing, falls and generalised weakness.

Cognitive and behavioural symptoms
People might report various symptoms involving cognition, personality and behaviour. Such symptoms might include overt personality change, aggression, agitation, irritability, memory loss, confusion, disorientation, lack of facial recognition, and disorders of thought including perceptual disturbances.

'John's Campaign' and extended visiting hours
'John's Campaign' is a movement to help NHS staff recognise the importance of working with family carers as equal partners in the care and support of people with a dementia who are in hospital.[21]

Carers in delirium can be potentially helpful in securing the diagnosis of delirium and in facilitating reality orientation in the subsequent management and recovery. Emergency and planned admissions to hospital are difficult experiences for any individual, but can be particularly traumatic for people with a delirium, often resulting in significant distress and deterioration of their condition. Often husbands, wives and significant others do not identify themselves as carers and don't really feel that this is what they are doing.

A 'carer's passport' can be useful to distinguish the carer from other visitors. This can be used to override restrictive visiting hours and initiate discussions between carers and ward managers about how best to plan care. John's Campaign advocates for carers to stay overnight should they wish as there may be times when this is crucial for the wellbeing of a person experiencing delirium.

It was hoped that extended visiting hours might result in reduced incidence and shorter length of delirium as well as shorter ICU stay. A 'flexible visiting policy' for family members in ICUs has been recommended by professional society guidelines as an important step toward patient- and family-centred care. Results from a recent study[22] suggest that, among patients in the ICU, a flexible family visiting policy did not significantly reduce the incidence of delirium compared with standard restricted visiting hours.

Regarding possible risks associated with flexible ICU visiting policies, some studies have shown that ICU professionals sometimes perceive visits as a source of increased workload and disorganisation in patient care.

Approach to the relief of symptoms

In addition to treating the underlying cause, management should also be directed at the relief of the symptoms of the delirium. The patient should be nursed in a good sensory environment and with a reality orientation approach, and with involvement of the multidisciplinary team. Communication with the relative regarding the nature of the delirium is essential. Depending on the layout and nature of the ward, these measures may be facilitated by nursing the patient in a single room, and facilitating 'reality orientation' of the patient. For example, in a busy ward, a patient with delirium may be better managed in a 'side room', whereas in a ward with small bays the presence of other patients may have a reassuring influence.

Potential components of 'good' person-centred care in delirium are shown in Box 4.1.

BOX 4.1 POTENTIAL COMPONENTS OF 'GOOD' PERSON-CENTRED DELIRIUM CARE

- Appropriate lighting levels for time of day
- Regular and repeated cues to improve personal orientation, use of clocks and calendars to improve orientation
- Reorientation to current news events
- Hearing aids, dentures and glasses available as appropriate and in good working order
- Removal of ear wax
- Continuity of care from nursing staff/familiar staff
- Encouragement of mobility and engagement in activities with other people
- Patient approached and handled gently
- Elimination of unexpected and irritating noise

- Regular analgesia, such as paracetamol
- Rationalisation of medication
- Encouragement of visits from family and friends who may be able to help calm the patient
- Explanation of the cause of the confusion to relatives
- Encouraging family to bring in familiar objects and pictures from home and to participate in cognitive rehabilitation
- Fluid intake to prevent dehydration
- Good diet
- Consider supplementary oxygen
- Good sleep hygiene
- Good lighting levels
- Stratification of 'falls risk'
- Reassurance and explanation to the patient and carer of any procedures or treatment, using short simple sentences
- Checking that the patient has understood you and being prepared to repeat if necessary
- Sensory aids available and working, where necessary
- Attending to bowel and bladder continence
- Extended visiting hours

Potential things to avoid in 'poor' person-centred care in delirium are shown in Box 4.2.

BOX 4.2 POTENTIAL 'THINGS TO AVOID' IN POOR CARE

- Inter- and intra-ward transfers
- Use of physical restraint
- Constipation and faecal impaction
- Arguments or confrontation
- Unnecessary procedures
- Anticholinergic drugs where possible, and keep drug treatment to a minimum
- Catheters where possible

Polypharmacy for people with delirium

A lack of time, knowledge or due diligence can also mean clinicians fail to recognise new symptoms as something caused by an older person's medication, rather than a deterioration of their condition(s).[23] True polypharmacy is defined as the use of several different medications by one patient at the same time. There are a number of individual and system factors which contribute to 'medication-related harm' when a person enters and leaves hospital.[24] Although polypharmacy can occur in both primary and secondary care, it is GPs who often take on the management of long-term conditions and prescriptions. A 'medication creep' occurs when clinicians fail to de-prescribe – or stop – medicines that an older person no longer needs or is no longer benefiting from.

Physical restraints

In the UK, physical restraints should be used when in the best interests of the patient, but some people dispute whether this is actually ever true in a patient with delirium. Physical restraints should be avoided whenever possible, as they lead to decreased mobility, increased agitation and risk of injury, sometimes resulting in death. Adequately staffing hospital units and providing optimal patient-care settings with frequent human interactions may assist in this regard. Minimal noise at night to allow an uninterrupted period of sleep at night is considered of crucial importance in the management of delirium.

The legal and ethical considerations of restraints are considered further in Chapter 10.

Family-centred care

It's essential to think of anyone known to the patient as an invaluable resource about that patient. Patient-centred care has been an important part of medicine since the 1970s; however, inclusion of the patient's family in care has recently grown in popularity. The relative 'invisibility' of the family in documentation and inconsistent levels of family inclusion in actual care act as barriers to enacting the team's voiced value of placing the person at the centre of care.

Family-centred care is the view that members of the patient's family are central members of the care team and also have needs themselves. Family can also help the staff, by assisting communication with the patient and by helping the patient interpret the environment through reorientation strategies, using personal objects and eyeglasses/hearing aids. They can also help to establish the initial diagnosis itself as an abrupt change in the patient's behaviour. When the family is involved in care, there is scope for more satisfaction and reassurance. Family members often represent the interests of their relatives and speak on their behalf when they are unable to express themselves comprehensibly. Nurses are ideally placed to respond compassionately to all members of the family, and provide appropriate reassurance, support and information during delirium. Information should include possible impacts on family and useful coping strategies.

The value of relationships

Relationship-centred care originally arose from discussions of a Task Force on health professions' curricula in the USA in the early 1990s. The phrase 'relationship-centred care' captures the importance of the interaction among people as the foundation of any therapeutic or teaching activity. Further, relationships are critical to the care provided by nearly all practitioners and a sense of satisfaction and positive outcomes for patients and practitioners.

The **senses framework** was developed by Nolan and colleagues[25] who proposed that six evidence-based senses underpin the notion of relationship-centred care, namely:

- security – to feel safe

- belonging – to feel part of things

- continuity – to experience links and connections

- purpose – to have a goal(s) to aspire to

- achievement – to make progress towards these goals

- significance – to feel that you matter as a person.

Goals

There are many factors which mitigate against acute hospital settings meeting the needs of people with cognitive impairment.

'Belonging'

While getting to know the anxieties, fears and needs of the individual is key to meeting the needs of the person with delirium, this is difficult in acute settings where lengths of stay tend to be short and there are significant time pressures. This can make it difficult for nurses to establish a good therapeutic relationship with the person, and can cause distress to the individual.

The role of specialist units and 'delirium rooms'

Modern hospice and palliative care units emerged in the 1960s with the opening of St Christopher's Hospice in London. A **'delirium unit'** or room can provide a calm, comfortable environment, which is helpful for agitated patients. In reality, patients with palliative care needs are located throughout hospital and community settings and have various life-threatening illnesses and other comorbidities.

'Delirium rooms' provide restraint-free care for patients with delirium, are staffed with specially trained nurses, and promote non-pharmacological management approaches.

The individuality of people with delirium

The contemporary focus on person-centredness in practice illustrates a drive away from fragmented disease-based approaches to holistic person-orientated approaches. This could present huge challenges to delirium care internationally. The challenge of delivering effective person-centred care, however, is often in the *translation* and detail. Person-centred care can provide insights into the experiences of the person with delirium and support care approaches and solutions to meet individual needs.

Person-centred practice requires healthcare professionals to **put the person first** and the evidence base for technical or clinical interventions second. Putting the person first requires expertise, and there still tends to be a lack of expert gerontological practitioners.

How a person-centred culture might catalyse person-centred care

What will really help catalysing a person-centred culture is credible management and leadership instilling credible beliefs and attitudes, such as viewing patients as persons with meaningful distinct lives.[26]

Ward-based staff can be supported to develop further communication skills to facilitate interaction with patients experiencing delirium and their relatives and any carers present. Further research is required, co-produced in partnership with patients who have experienced delirium, and their carers, to explore their experience. Understanding this is essential to ensuring that their opinions are identified, valued, respected and incorporated into the commissioning of future acute healthcare services.

There is an urgent need to 'pull' delirium care away from the ethos of a 'production line' – as Professor Ed Schein says:[27]

To describe the process of getting from that role-based transaction to this more personal relationship we're coining the word personize – not personalize, but personize. Get to know each other in the work context… We're not building an assembly line or a nice model factory. We're struggling with complex issues that don't resolve easily.

Endnotes

1   Grealish, L., Chaboyer, W., Mudge, A., Simpson, T. et al. (2019) 'Using a general theory of implementation to plan the introduction of delirium prevention in older people in hospital.' Journal of Nursing Management 27, 8, 1631–1639. Accessed on 29/11/2019 at www.ncbi.nlm.nih.gov/pubmed/31444812.

2   Garand, L., Lingler, J.H., Conner, K.O. and Dew, M.A. (2009) 'Diagnostic labels, stigma, and participation in research related to dementia and mild cognitive impairment.' Research in Gerontological Nursing 2, 2, 112–121. Accessed on 29/11/2019 at www.ncbi.nlm.nih.gov/pmc/articles/PMC2864081.

3   British Geriatrics Society (2019) 'Are "frailty units" and "dementia wards" the anathema of pure person-centred care?' Accessed on 29/11/2019 at www.bgs.org.uk/blog/are-'frailty-units'-and-'dementia-wards'-the-anathema-of-pure-person-centred-care.

4   Ben Malek, H., Philippi, N., Botzung, A., Cretin, B. et al. (2019) 'Memories defining the self in Alzheimer's disease.' Memory 27, 5, 698–704. Accessed on 29/11/2019 at www.ncbi.nlm.nih.gov/pubmed/30526307.

5   Farzanegan, B., Elkhatib, T.H.M., Elgazzar, A.E., Moghaddam, K.G. et al. (2019) 'Impact of religiosity on delirium severity among critically ill Shi'a Muslims: A prospective multi-center observational study.' Journal of Religion and Health. Accessed on 29/11/2019 at https://link.springer.com/article/10.1007/s10943-019-00895-7.

6   Davis, D., Searle, S.D. and Tsui, A. (2019) 'The Scottish Intercollegiate Guidelines Network: Risk reduction and management of delirium.' Age and Ageing 48, 4, 485–488. Accessed on 29/11/2019 at www.ncbi.nlm.nih.gov/pubmed/30927352.

7   Teodorczuk, A., Mukaetova-Ladinska, E., Corbett, S. and Welfare, M. (2015) 'Deconstructing dementia and delirium hospital practice: Using cultural historical activity theory to inform education approaches.' Advances in Health Sciences Education: Theory and Practice 20, 3, 745–764. Accessed on 29/11/2019 at www.ncbi.nlm.nih.gov/pubmed/25354660.

8   Welch, C. and Jackson, T.A. (2018) 'Can delirium research activity impact on routine delirium recognition? A prospective cohort study.' BMJ Open 8, e0123386. Accessed on 29/11/2019 at https://bmjopen.bmj.com/content/8/10/e023386.

9   Carucci, R. (2019) 'Leading change in a company that's historically bad at it.' Harvard Business Review, 6 August. Accessed on 29/11/2019 at https://hbr.org/2019/08/leading-change-in-a-company-thats-historically-bad-at-it.

10   Koren, M.J. (2010) 'Person-centered care for nursing home residents: The culture-change movement.' Health Affairs 29, 2, 312–317. Accessed on 29/11/2019 at www.healthaffairs.org/doi/10.1377/hlthaff.2009.0966.

11   Quality Care Commission (2019) 'Regulation 9: Person-centred care.' Accessed on 29/11/2019 at www.cqc.org.uk/guidance-providers/regulations-enforcement/regulation-9-person-centred-care.

12   Young, J. and Inouye, S.K. (2007) 'Delirium in older people.' BMJ 334, 7598, 842–846. Accessed on 16/12/2019 at www.ncbi.nlm.nih.gov/pmc/articles/PMC1853193.

13   Parsons, T., Tregunno, M.J., Joneja, M., Dalgarno, N. and Flynn, L. (2018) 'Using graphic illustrations to uncover how a community of practice can influence the delivery of compassionate healthcare.' Medical Humanities. Accessed on 29/11/2019 at https://mh.bmj.com/content/early/2018/09/26/medhum-2018-011508.

14   Borgstrom, E. (2017) 'Social death.' QJM: Monthly Journal of the Association of Physicians 110, 1, 5–7. Accessed on 29/11/2019 at www.ncbi.nlm.nih.gov/pubmed/27770051.

15   Tinetti, M.E. and Fried, T. (2004) 'The end of the disease era.' American Journal of Medicine 116, 3, 179–185. Accessed on 29/11/2019 at www.amjmed.com/article/S0002-9343(03)00666-1/abstract.

16   Age UK (2019) 'Later Life in the United Kingdom 2019.' Accessed on 29/11/2019 at www.ageuk.org.uk/globalassets/age-uk/documents/reports-and-publications/later_life_uk_factsheet.pdf.

17   NHS Commissioning Board (2012) *Compassion in Practice: Nursing, Midwifery and Care Staff. Our Vision and Strategy*. Leeds: Department of Health. Accessed on 29/11/2019 at www.england.nhs.uk/wp-content/uploads/2012/12/compassion-in-practice.pdf.

18   Collier, A., De Bellis, A., Hosie, A., Dadich, A. *et al.* (2019) 'Fundamental care for people with cognitive impairment in a hospital setting: A study combining positive organisational scholarship and video-reflexive ethnography.' *Journal of Clinical Nursing*. Accessed on 29/11/2019 at www.ncbi.nlm.nih.gov/pubmed/31495005.

19   van der Cingel, M., Brandsma, L., van Dam, M., van Dorst, M., Verkaart, C. and van der Velde, C. (2016) 'Concepts of person-centred care: A framework analysis of five studies in daily care practice.' *International Practice Development Journal 6*, 2, 6. Accessed on 29/11/2019 at www.fons.org/library/journal/volume6-issue2/article6.

20   Davydow, D.S. (2009) 'Symptoms of depression and anxiety after delirium.' *Psychosomatics 50*, 4, 309–316.

21   Gold Standards Framework (2015) 'John's Campaign – Dementia.' Accessed on 29/11/2019 at www.goldstandardsframework.org.uk/john-s-campaign-dementia.

22   Rosa, R.G., Falavigna, M., da Silva, D.B., Sganzeria, D. *et al.* (2019) 'Effect of flexible family visitation on delirium among patients in the intensive care unit: The ICU visits randomized clinical trial.' *JAMA 322*, 3, 216–228. Accessed on 29/11/2019 at www.ncbi.nlm.nih.gov/pubmed/31310297.

23   Age UK (2019) 'More harm than good.' Accessed on 29/11/2019 at www.ageuk.org.uk/globalassets/age-uk/documents/reports-and-publications/reports-and-briefings/health--wellbeing/medication/190819_more_harm_than_good.pdf.

24   Parekh, N., Ali, K., Davies, J.G., Stevenson, J.M. *et al.* (2019) 'Medication-related harm in older adults following hospital discharge: Development and validation of a prediction tool.' *BMJ Quality and Safety*. Accessed on 29/11/2019 at https://qualitysafety.bmj.com/content/early/2019/09/16/bmjqs-2019-009587.

25   Nolan, M., Brown, J., Davies, S., Nolan, J. and Keady, J. (2006) *The SENSES Framework: Improving Care for Older People Through a Relationship-Centred Approach*. Sheffield: University of Sheffield.

26   Kambil, A. (2019) 'Catalyzing organizational culture change.' *Deloitte Insights*. Accessed on 29/11/2019 at www2.deloitte.com/insights/us/en/focus/executive-transitions/organizational-culture-change.html.

27   Zehnder, E. (2019) 'In conversation with Ed Schein.' Accessed on 29/11/2019 at www.egonzehnder.com/insight/in-conversation-with-ed-schein.

5

Communication, interaction and behaviour in delirium care

LEARNING OBJECTIVES

Communication can be non-verbal as well as verbal. Compassionate and effective communication and interactions between people lie at the heart of clinical care, and there is a regulatory obligation for clinicians to provide good communication at all times. Communication might be between the patient with delirium and care staff, but it might also be between clinicians themselves. You'll consider the particular importance of communication in delirium care in this chapter.

Introduction

It is essential to communicate the diagnosis to patients and carers, encourage involvement of carers and provide ongoing engagement and support. A lack of communication and the need for healthcare staff to be more communicative about delirium has been identified in studies in non-ICU settings.[1]

Good communication with family members or carers is crucial. Family members can provide background information on patient history, changes in personality and behaviour, and 'early warning signs'.

Once the diagnosis of delirium is made, carers need information and support to enable them to care for the patient. Communication is pervasive to this ethical care, and might include, for example, responding to the non-verbal communication of the patient, and liaising between the patient and family.

Communication in delirium

Box 5.1 suggests ways to support communication.

BOX 5.1 SUPPORTING COMMUNICATION

- Listen in a calm, gentle, friendly, affectionate and reassuring manner.
- Use verbal and non-verbal ways of reassuring.
- Keep a calendar or clock within view.
- Make the patient feel as if he is in control.
- Address pain by looking for non-verbal signs of pain, particularly in those with communication difficulties.
- Avoid arguing.
- Do not insist that the person experiencing delirium is wrong or unreasonable. Be tactful, or change the subject.
- Try to understand and meet the person's emotional needs.
- Try to remember that the person is not being deliberately difficult; don't take it personally.
- 'Understanding' the person and their history will help.
- Familiarity helps, so try to make sure that someone the patient knows well is with them.
- Consider whether the behaviour is really a problem.
- Check that tests for any sensory impairments are up to date.
- Remind the patient to eat and drink regularly.
- Ensure any dentures are fitted.
- Ensure any sensory aids are fitted.

Any distressed behaviour may be a response to the person feeling that they are not able to contribute or are not valued by others.

The importance of effective communication in delirium care

Communication is a complex process, which involves much emotional intelligence. Effective coordination and communication between the individual, their family and the healthcare professionals involved are necessary.

Patient-centred communication is a key part of care. Important skills include eliciting patients' and families' perspectives in an open-ended fashion, listening and observing all cues, and responding to emotions with empathy. Optimal delirium management requires good interprofessional communication, but, with current pressures in the workforce, all individuals presently often have little time to communicate with each other.

Communication between patients and practitioners lies at the heart of delirium healthcare.

It is important to consider that communication:

- can enhance diagnostic accuracy and reliability, promote patient-centred treatment decisions and improve a number of clinical outcomes ranging from treatment adherence to safety

- is challenging, but is possible to do very well and it is worthwhile

- should include simple language expressed in a clearly audible, slow-paced voice.

We need to learn from failures too. 'Self-reflection' also permits physicians to step back from a conversation with the patient and family, and reflect on issues such as how his or her own emotions might influence decision-making for the patient. Nobody is infallible, and there is always scope to do things better and to learn from experience.

Types of communication

Communication refers to 'exchanges' between individuals and social interactions. We tend to think of communication as only speaking and listening, but in fact it consists of much more than that. As much as 90% of our communication takes place through non-verbal communication such as gestures, facial expression and touch. Non-verbal communication is particularly important for a person with dementia who may be losing their language skills. When a person with dementia behaves in ways that cause problems for their carer, and appears 'distressed', he might be trying to communicate something as crucial as pain.

Components of non-verbal communication

We all communicate through facial expressions, body language, gestures and touch. Non-verbal communication is important and provides clues about how someone is feeling and what they are trying to communicate. Picking up on cues may be especially important in the case in delirium where verbal communication can border on 'gibberish'.

Posture
Posture is a part of body language and gives an indication of whether the person with you is interested, sick or has a sensory impairment, among other things. The ideal is 'non-threatening posture' from clinicians.

Facial expressions
Facial expressions tell us what people are thinking even when they do not realise it. Sometimes even what we say is contradicted by what our body language is saying. It's thought to be hard to 'fake' facial expressions.

Eye contact
Eye contact is essential for social and emotional cognition. Lack of eye contact and looking disinterested are obvious barriers to communication.

Appropriate use of touch and personal space
Touch or contact can be very comforting, but you must be careful to use touch respectfully and appropriately.

Gestures
Gestures are signals our body uses to convey messages.

Communication difficulties of people with delirium
Studies on communication difficulties in patients experiencing delirium have reported significant issues when conveying basic information, as reported by patients, their relatives and nursing staff. Yet relatively few studies have investigated the nature of language abnormalities in actual patients in delirium. Fundamental domains of language such as speech production in delirium have been unexplored, but a study has reported language impairments in over half of patients with delirium.[2] Speech content and verbal and written language comprehension are both said to be impaired in patients with delirium compared with cognitively unimpaired patients.[3]

Efficient communication between a clinician and a patient is essential for effective management of pain, nutrition and hydration, which are a common concern in people with delirium. With regard to communicating with patients experiencing delirium in clinical care, the diverse range of impairments seen in delirium highlight the need for communication strategies adapted to the respective needs of patients and delirium-focused communication guidelines.

Rambling speech

Patients with delirium often exhibit confused and rambling speech. It is usually preferable not to agree with 'rambling talk', but to adopt one of the following strategies, depending on the circumstance:

- tactfully disagree (if the topic is not sensitive)

- change the subject

- acknowledge the feelings expressed while ignoring the content.

Because of communication difficulties, it can be extremely difficult to elicit ideas, concerns and expectations as you might to do for most people about their illnesses.

The need for high-quality information

A valuable goal is to train healthcare staff to help facilitate open discussions with patients about their *personal experience* of delirium (see Chapter 9), and to supervise clinicians to allow patients to understand better – and manage – their own anxieties. Knowledge is power.

Communication in all care settings represents a reciprocal partnership between many parties. Communication must be responsive to the needs in an individual encounter, but the encounter should be person-centred rather than simply transactional. Clinicians need information about delirium to alleviate their insecurity about interactions with the patient and to aid their understanding of the patient's behaviour which will allow trust to develop. Providing essential, relevant and clear information for patients and relatives, even in an information factsheet, to help them understand delirium can be beneficial. Once diagnosed, carers need information and support for their care for the patient in the actual present and in the future. It is necessary to inform relatives of the short-term nature of delirium, and the willingness to offer support and advice from professionals on how to communicate. Here, estimating prognosis is an unpleasant area for delirium clinicians. For example:

> While receiving prognostic information is difficult for patients, not receiving prognostic information can create anxiety and may distance patients from their clinicians, who are often aware of the prognosis but do not share it with patients. Delaying or avoiding communication about prognosis also risks patients not having the information they need to make decisions and leads to missed opportunities to set and achieve goals that reflect what matters most to them.[4]

Communication is nevertheless a key element of the delirium 'lived experience':

- being in the delirium

- responding to delirium

- dealing with delirium.

Active listening skills

Active listening is an effective level of listening, and it is a specialist skill. It is based on complete attention to what a person is saying, listening carefully while showing interest and not interrupting. Active listening can help to improve communication between you and the person you're caring for.

Active listening includes:

- using eye contact to look at the person, and encouraging them to look at you when either of you are talking

- a calm and friendly manner

- listening for the content, intent and feeling of the speaker

- trying not to interrupt

- stopping what you're doing so you can give the person your full attention while they speak

- finding a peaceful setting if possible

- repeating what you heard back to the person and asking if it's accurate, or asking them to repeat what they said

- avoiding confrontation, contradiction or humiliation.

The importance of speaking clearly, calmly and with patience
Speak clearly

Speak clearly, calmly and slowly to allow the person time to understand information. Use simple, short sentences. Keep choices to a minimum and don't raise your voice. Where possible, talk in a noise free, non-distracting place or find a quiet corner.

Body language

People with cognitive difficulties may find it difficult to understand what is being said, but can be quick to interpret the message on people's faces and may still be aware of body language.

Smile warmly, make eye contact, make sure you are at the person's level and use a friendly tone.

Show respect and patience

Adapt what you are saying if the person does not understand. Don't rush.

Listen

Listen carefully to what the person is trying to say, giving plenty of encouragement even if it sounds like nonsense.

Talk to the person

Automatically going to talk to their partner or carer and ignoring or not including the person can be very upsetting and feel really undermining.

Recommendations,[5] especially in communication with patients who are psychotic, refer to "'open hands, open gestures'", and refraining from any gestures associated with ordering, commanding, hierarchy and authoritarianism, such as: "wagging your finger", "staring people out", "pointing at people", "folding arms" and "standing with hands on your hips".

Supply fully functioning sensory aids

A number of people with delirium will have some form of sensory impairment (such as sight loss, hearing loss or both), and aids to address these impairments must be provided.

Social cognitive difficulties

Hyperactive delirium on the face of it looks to be a disorder of empathy, among many things. Empathy is a multidimensional construct consisting of cognitive (inferring mental states) and emotional (understanding people's intentions and feelings) components.[6] Social communication difficulties are strongly associated with injury to the anterior frontal lobes of the brain.

Other potential wider problems with social cognition may include:

- interrupting someone else because they are afraid that otherwise they will forget what they want to say

- speaking only about themselves and fixating on certain subjects
- talking in a disinhibited way
- getting stuck on individual words, topics or themes
- altered ability to give information in an orderly and organised way
- not using or 'reading' non-verbal cues accurately, such as facial expressions and body language.

Sensory problems
Hearing loss
How a person with hearing loss communicates will depend on a range of factors including the type of hearing loss they have and whether they use a hearing aid, British Sign Language,[7] lip-reading or a combination of all of them. But there are important gaps in our knowledge here – we do not know whether deaf patients experiencing delirium are able to lip-read.

Sight loss
Many people experience some degree of sight loss as they get older. Not being able to see what is around them can lead to yet further disorientation and distress, as well as decreased mobility and a risk of falls. Having both delirium and sight loss can also make people feel isolated from those around them.

How life-story information may enable or support more effective communication
For people with a cognitive impairment, however, the link between past and present life events can become disconnected. Clinicians often express the belief that increased personal knowledge of the patient with cognitive impairment can improve the hospital experience for all. The telling of a chronological life story, however, becomes challenged as a result of various cognitive effects, especially through impairments in autobiographical and memory functioning.

Benefits of a 'life-story approach' include enhanced wellbeing improvements in mood and some domains of cognition, and improvements in confidence and social interaction.

Not knowing the patient's former personality or life story can be significant factor negatively influencing the relationship between the clinician and patient. Knowledge of patients' life stories can guide nurses to care for specific interests of patients experiencing delirium.

Agitation

The study of complex behaviours in persons with neurodegenerative conditions is difficult. Discussing treatment of agitation in Alzheimer's disease, Howard reports:[8]

> Given the complexity of the symptoms and behaviors and their individual etiology, involving patient-unique interactions between an impaired brain and an imperfect environment, it should come as no surprise when trials report only modest benefits that, when considered for the average participant in the study, would not be regarded as clinically important.

For people in hospital and other care settings, agitation is a major problem. Distressed behaviours have been framed as an active attempt by the person to express an unfulfilled need, which could be physiological or psychological. Agitation might be a manifestation of distress or suffering, or a reaction to something done by a carer, which may in turn exacerbate communication problems. Before any rational intervention can be formulated, especially one respecting dignity and other human rights, the distressed behaviour needs to be properly identified, understood and evaluated; for this, a person-centred approach is essential.

In the real world, the running of medical wards can be handicapped by a poor nurse-to-patient ratio, particularly during night shifts when agitation occurs more often.

Agitation is, arguably, also a symptom of much wider system factors at play.

Rather than see the behaviour as a problem, it should be seen as a method of communication. What is the person trying to tell us? Failure to do this results in people with distressed behaviour being branded 'problem patients'.

It is nonetheless essential to acknowledge that an agitated patient with delirium could pose a danger to himself or herself and hospital staff. The top priority here in management of this patient is safety. The patient should be temporarily placed in a safe area, and non-pharmacological intervention should be instituted first.

The first recommended non-pharmacological intervention is verbal de-escalation of the situation. Signs such as changes in tone and speed of speech, irritability, pacing and clenched fist or jaw all indicate that this method of intervention is insufficient. However, sometimes agitation care is not particularly person-centred.[9]

Communication of the delirium diagnosis with GPs

NICE Quality statement 5: Communication of diagnosis to GPs states: 'Adults with current or resolved delirium who are discharged from hospital have their diagnosis of delirium communicated to their GP.'[10]

Improving communication between various clinical stakeholders may help people who are recovering from or who still have delirium to receive adequate follow-up care on hospital discharge. Follow-up care may include treatment for reversible causes, investigation for possible dementia and a greater emphasis on preventing delirium recurring.

A person's diagnosis of delirium may not be communicated to their GP because it is usually secondary to their main reason for admission, and it also may not be communicated between hospital wards when the person is transferred.

A person's diagnosis of delirium during a hospital stay should be formally included in the discharge summary sent to their GP, and the term 'delirium' should be used.

Endnotes

1   O'Malley, G., Leonard, M., Meagher, D. and O'Keeffe, S.T. (2008) 'The delirium experience.' *Journal of Psychosomatic Research 65*, 3, 223–228. Accessed on 29/11/2019 at www.ncbi.nlm.nih.gov/pubmed/18707944.

2   Green, S., Reivonen, S., Rutter, L.-M., Nouzova, E. *et al.* (2018) 'Investigating speech and language impairments in delirium: A preliminary case-control study.' *PLOS One 13*, 11, e0207527. Accessed on 29/11/2019 at www.ncbi.nlm.nih.gov/pmc/articles/PMC6261049.

3   Green, S., Reivonen, S., Rutter, L.-M., Nouzova, E. *et al.* (2018) 'Investigating speech and language impairments in delirium: A preliminary case-control study.' *PLOS One 13*, 11, e0207527. Accessed on 29/11/2019 at www.ncbi.nlm.nih.gov/pmc/articles/PMC6261049.

4   Paladino, J., Lakin, J.R. and Sanders, J.J. (2019) 'Communication strategies for sharing prognostic information with patients: Beyond survival statistics.' *JAMA 322*, 14, 1345–1346. Accessed on 29/11/2019 at https://jamanetwork.com/journals/jama/fullarticle/2748666.

5   Bowers, L., Brennan, G., Winship, G. and Theodoridou, C. (2009) 'Communication skills for nurses and others spending time with people who are very mentally ill.' Accessed on 29/11/2019 at www.kcl.ac.uk/ioppn/depts/hspr/archive/mhn/projects/Talking.pdf.

6   Dziobek, I., Rogers, K., Fleck, S. Bahnemann, M. *et al.* (2008) 'Dissociation of cognitive and emotional empathy in adults with Asperger syndrome using the Multifaceted Empathy Test (MET).' *Journal of Autism and Developmental Disorders 38*, 3, 464–473. Accessed on 29/11/2019 at www.ncbi.nlm.nih.gov/pubmed/17990089.

7   See www.british-sign.co.uk.

8   Howard, R.J. (2016) 'Disentangling the treatment of agitation in Alzheimer's disease.' *American Journal of Psychiatry 173*, 5, 441–443. Accessed on 29/11/2019 at https://ajp.psychiatryonline.org/doi/full/10.1176/appi.ajp.2016.16010083?url_ver=Z39.88-2003&rfr_id=ori:rid:crossref.org&rfr_dat=cr_pub%3dpubmed.

9   Pritchard, J.C. and Brighty, A. (2015) 'Caring for older people experiencing agitation.' *Nursing Standard* 29, 30, 49–58. Accessed on 29/11/2019 at www.ncbi.nlm.nih.gov/pubmed/25804179.

10   NICE Quality statement 5: Communication of diagnosis to GPs. Quality standard [QS63] Published date: July 2014. Accessed on 29/11/2019 at www.nice.org.uk/guidance/qs63/chapter/quality-statement-5-communication-of-diagnosis-to-gps.

6

Health and wellbeing in delirium

LEARNING OBJECTIVES

High-quality delirium care is high-quality care across many domains, including mobilisation, nutrition and hydration. As such, it might seem odd that these should be given particular consideration in delirium. But patients experiencing delirium are often at high risk because of their background and outcomes. In this chapter, you'll be invited to consider aspects of health and wellbeing to be promoted prior to and at the time of the onset of delirium across a variety of care settings.

Introduction

The importance for individuals to maintain good physical and mental health before, during and after the delirious event is pivotal. In delirium care, there is an overall need to optimise physiology, management of concurrent conditions, environment, medications and natural sleep, to promote good 'brain health'.

Anticipating an individual's health needs

Aspects of healthy living can include:

- physiotherapy

- reorientation

- early mobilisation

- identification and treatment of underlying causes or post-operative complications

- pain control

- regulation of bowel and bladder function

- hydration and nutrition

- oxygen delivery.

Comprehensive geriatric care, including comprehensive medical assessment,[1] helps greatly with delirium care.

Sleep

There is a strong relationship between sleep abnormalities and cognitive disorders. Sleep disturbances can present as insomnia, abnormalities in sleep architecture, daytime somnolence, and reversal of sleep–wake phases, and are measurable for example using the Delirium Rating Scale-Revised-98.[2]

An obvious point: if possible, don't disturb a patient's sleep with procedures and medication rounds.

> **ADVICE GIVEN TO PATIENTS**
> Good sleep could help protect you from delirium. Sleep can be difficult in hospital, but an eye mask or ear plugs may help. If you don't have any, ask a nurse. Try to avoid caffeinated drinks in the evening.

Nutrition and hydration

It is biologically plausible that many disease conditions lead to specific physiological abnormalities in the cerebral cortex. These conditions include metabolic disorders and abnormal nutrition and hydration. Micronutrient deficiencies in mineral and trace elements, antioxidants and other vitamin deficiencies such as B_{12} status are mooted to impact on delirium onset.

> **ADVICE GIVEN TO PATIENTS**
> Drinking and eating enough is important to prevent delirium. If you need dentures, please ensure you have them. Discuss your fluid intake with a doctor or nurse if you have heart or kidney failure.

Mobilisation, socialisation and keeping active

Early mobilisation is good practice.

Physical function is affected by chronic diseases in adults and older patients.

Bed rest has been associated with a number of unfortunate sequelae, including, not least, 'undesirable cardiovascular, pulmonary and urinary effects, reduced muscle tone, loss of bone mineral density, and negative psychological effects'.[3]

Short-term bed rest typically occurs during hospitalisation for an acute disease or delirium, and is a major contributor to functional decline in older adults. Studies, for example, have indicated that reductions in muscle tissue following bed rest or immobilisation may be driven by a slower muscle protein synthesis rate at rest.[4]

Physical activity is universally recognised to have positive health benefits and has been associated with improved cognitive function and brain health.[5]

A recent systematic review and meta-analysis of published randomised controlled trials found significant improvements in walking speed as a measure of fitness among those who took part in programmes to encourage mobilisation, compared with patients who did not.[6]

Occupational therapy is defined by the World Federation of Occupational Therapists as a 'profession concerned with promoting health and wellbeing through occupation'.[7] Occupational therapists try to achieve this goal helping the patient reach optimal capacity to participate in these activities, and/or by modifying the environment so that it is easier for his participation to take place.

It is also considered advantageous to encourage *socialisation* as well as mobilisation. One recommendation is to engage the patient in conversation while mobilising, and encourage the patient to talk with others while walking in the corridor.[8] Another has to been to encourage socialisation in 'mealtimes'.[9]

ADVICE GIVEN TO PATIENTS

Try to stay mobile – this is especially important after surgery. You may be able to walk about or do mobility exercises.

Medication review

All patients at risk of delirium should have a medication review conducted by an experienced healthcare professional.

Delirium has numerous causes that interact in any one person to cause delirium.

Several classes of medication can increase the likelihood of delirium occurring, and the probability that a drug will precipitate delirium should be considered when prescribing, particularly in those already at increased risk of delirium due to predisposing factors.

Medication reviews are part of the national and international guidelines for the prevention and management of delirium in hospital patients. However, it has been argued[10] that these guidelines are not common practice for all older patients.

The following is suggested[11] by SIGN as an approach to medication review and prescribing in people who are experiencing, or are at increased risk of, delirium, and covers three broad areas:

- any changes in medications, including over-the-counter and herbal medications

- changes in how the body handles and is affected by medication

- delirium risk should be considered when assessing the risks and benefits of commencing a new medication.

For people at risk of delirium, a systematic review[12] mentioned that opioids should be prescribed with caution in people at risk of delirium, bearing in mind that untreated severe pain can itself trigger delirium.

Continence
Regulation of bladder and bowel function
Continence interventions can reduce or minimise functional decline and promote social continence and good bladder habits and strategies.

The environment can make it difficult for a person to access the toilet, so it is worth seeking to modify the environment so the person can go to the toilet independently. An individualised continence management plan could be developed and implemented in conjunction with the older person and a multidisciplinary team. It should be regularly reviewed and adjusted as needed.

Some useful suggestions are given below:[13]

- Orientate the person to where the 'call bell' is.

- Orientate the person to where the toilet is.

- Consider moving the person to a bed closer to the toilet.

- Provide adequate lighting.

- Consider altering the person's clothing to make using a toilet easier.

Breathing
Provision of supplementary oxygen, if appropriate
When a person isn't getting enough oxygen, all organs of the body can be affected, especially the brain, heart and kidneys.

A fall in oxygen perfusion of the brain is thought to compromise levels of consciousness, and depressed consciousness often leads to airway obstruction leading to further problems.

Prevention of complications
Aim to prevent complications of delirium, which include:

- falls

- pressure sores

- immobility

- dehydration

- social isolation and loneliness

- nosocomial infections

- functional impairment

- continence problems

- over-sedation

- malnutrition.

Problems in nutrition, hydration and feeding
Under-nutrition clearly impacts on the quality of care in all settings. Older adults might not be focused on nutrition and hydration. As a population, elder patients might have many limitations that may contribute to weight loss and nutritional problems.

The reasons for malnutrition are complex, for example:

- decreased functional status and dysphagia

- reduced food intake

- iatrogenic reasons for malnutrition including limited numbers of nursing assistants to help during meals, poor-quality food and polypharmacy

- abnormalities in homeostasis[14]
- a fear of incontinence.

Implications for clinical practice relate to the need for better nutritional assessment, especially those with delirium. Preventing malnutrition in susceptible individuals most likely will decrease the incidence of delirium and also improve clinical outcomes in other areas such as skin integrity.

Delirium is associated with unsafe swallow on admission. In delirium, some individuals simply stop drinking. A 'swallowing screening' in a multidisciplinary context could be considered helpful to rule out dysphagia.

Aspiration pneumonia can be a serious problem, often requiring transfer to a hospital and a lengthy stay there. It is associated with a high mortality rate and is very costly to healthcare systems. Delirium is a predictor of aspiration pneumonia in nursing-home residents.[15] Dysphagia has been identified as one of the most important risk factors for aspiration pneumonia.

Many people's swallowing abilities fluctuate, sometimes from hour to hour, and staff need to have, and be encouraged to use, common sense, experience and judgement in these circumstances.

Contemporary **risk-feeding policies**[16] may perpetuate common misperceptions that there is a straightforward relationship between aspiration and pneumonia and that interventions such as 'nil by mouth' or tube feeding will reduce the risk of pneumonia, and may reduce the potential for individualised and flexible decision-making.

Polypharmacy

Often, patients are prescribed with medications and no one reviews the need at a future date.

Diverse physiological changes in older unwell patients may influence drug pharmacokinetics and pharmacodynamics. Polypharmacy is common among critically ill older adults and is associated with increased adverse events, greater drug interactions and increased costs. There is a tremendous need for interdisciplinary collaboration between all specialists to prevent the phenomenon of polypharmacy.

There had been, thus far, a lack of consensus on the definition of **deprescribing**, but a relatively recent article proposed the following definition: 'Deprescribing is the process of withdrawal of an inappropriate medication, supervised by a health care professional with the goal of managing polypharmacy and improving outcomes.'[17]

All patients at risk of delirium should have a medication review conducted by an experienced healthcare professional at reasonable time intervals.

Falls

For those who fall, the risk of sustaining a fracture is three times higher than for cognitively well people.

Things to consider when a person falls:

- What is the blood pressure?

- Is there a reversible cause or is it related to another medical condition? Is the person taking multiple medications?

- Is the patient living with frailty? Is there an underlying mobility or balance problem?

- Is there an underlying cognitive or behavioural problem?

- Is there an underlying neurological problem such as Parkinson's disease?

- Is the person experiencing medication side effects or interactions? Are medications being taken as prescribed?

- Does the person have changes in vision or any other sensory impairment?

- Is the person in pain but unable to recognise or communicate their discomfort?

In the United States, since 2007, there has been a striking trend towards immobility among hospitalised older adults; according to a 2009 estimate, hospital patients spend over 95% of their time in bed.[18]

When older adults are hospitalised, there is an inherent tension between preventing falls and promoting mobility. Although falls with injury should, of course, be avoided in the hospital, current fall prevention efforts reflect an underlying assumption that keeping patients from moving altogether can stop such falls. It has been suggested that this issue requires cultural change: that fall prevention teams at hospitals could be transformed into mobility teams, and patient-centred outcome measures could include surveys eliciting patients' experiences with practices related to preventing falls and promoting mobility.[19]

Fall prevention can be encouraged by continuous auditing including re-education.[20]

It is particularly noteworthy that the Hospital Elder Life Program (HELP) has been found to be effective in reducing incidence of delirium and rate of falls, with a trend toward decreasing length of stay and preventing transfer to residential settings.[21]

Deconditioning

Deconditioning is the 'process of physiological change following a period of inactivity or bedrest that results in a decrease in muscle mass, weakness, functional decline and the inability to perform daily living activities',[22] accelerated in comparison with normal ageing.

Deconditioning in older hospitalised patients is consistently reported, more often due to hospitalisation rather than presenting medical illness. The most consistent and pronounced changes with bed rest include the rapid loss of lower extremity muscle mass.[23]

Complications

Inactivity and prolonged bed rest is an unnatural state of the human body. Complications include:

- osteoporosis

- cardiovascular changes

- respiratory

- skin changes (e.g. pressure ulcers)

- gastrointestinal changes (e.g. decreased appetite; constipation)

- psychosocial (e.g. depression, loss of independence, loss of motivation).

Preventing a 'deconditioning syndrome' requires a broader strategic approach that includes physical therapy, maintenance of nutrition and psychological support including addressing loneliness.

Possible ways forward are listed in Box 6.1.

BOX 6.1 AVOIDING DECONDITIONING

- Promote awareness.
- Ensure that patients are sitting up in chairs, preferably in their own clothes.
- Ensure that meals are eaten while sitting in chairs and not spoon-fed in bed unless circumstances dictate that spoon feeding is necessary.
- Encourage patients to wash and dress independently.
- Encourage patients to walk to the toilet where possible.
- Provide appropriate mobility aids earlier on.
- Ensure that the patient's chair and mobility aids are of the right height.
- Check whether the urinary catheter (if present) is still required.

If you're interested in these issues, it might be worth joining the 'End PJ Paralysis' movement.[24] The campaign aims to get older people back home to their loved ones living much happier and fuller lives.[25]

Signs and symptoms of poor nutrition and hydration

There are many ways to increase a person's appetite and interest in food and drink.

Swallowing difficulties (dysphagia) could be related to delirium, but equally could be due to dementia, stroke, abscesses, tumours or other degenerative conditions.

Some features of poor nutrition include:

- feeling tired all the time

- increased infections

- constipation

- lack of energy

- gaining or losing weight

- depression

- poor wound healing.

Recognition of dehydration can be challenging, as physical signs of dehydration have a poor sensitivity and specificity in older people in comparison with laboratory measures.

Some features of poor hydration include:

- feelings of thirst as the body tries to increase fluid levels
- dark-coloured urine as the body tries to reduce fluid loss
- headaches and fatigue
- poor wound healing
- kidney problems.

Individuals should have access to fluid at all times, unless it is restricted for medical reasons. They should be encouraged to drink throughout the day and not wait until they feel thirsty, as feelings of thirst are an early sign of dehydration.

Drinks need to be placed within easy reach for those with restricted movement or mobility.

Dehydration may indicate, at worst, substandard care, if it arises due to lack of shift time or even neglect.

Box 6.2 gives some ideas that may help in helping people to benefit from healthy eating.

BOX 6.2 HEALTHY EATING AND DELIRIUM

- Make food look and smell appealing. Use different tastes, colours and smells. The aroma of cooking can benefit appetite – e.g. the smell of freshly baked bread.
- Look for opportunities to encourage the person to eat.
- Give the person food they like. Try not to overload the plate with too much food – small and regular portions often work best.
- Try different types of food or drinks.
- If food goes cold, it will lose its appeal. Cold food should therefore be reheated in a timely and efficient way where possible.
- If you do consider pureed food, seek advice from a dietitian and/or speech and language therapist.

How to recognise and manage pain in people with delirium

Persistent pain can lead to decreased mobility. It can also have a marked effect on cognition and behaviour.

People with a delirium can experience both physical and psychological pain but may not express this in conventional ways.

If a person becomes aggressive or agitated because of pain, they may be prescribed inappropriate medications which potentially have serious adverse effects. Treating the underlying pain should alleviate the resulting problem behaviours.

It also can be difficult for clinicians to administer and interpret pain assessment instruments.

In patients on the ICU, who are known to have especially high rates of delirium, mechanical ventilation and sedation can make assessment of pain through self-report tricky.

Adequate pain control is very important.

Supporting an individual in maintaining personal appearance and hygiene

A person's appearance is integral to their self-respect, and older people need to receive appropriate levels of support to maintain the standards they are used to. Personal preferences should be respected, as well as choice in how support is provided. For example, choosing when and how to carry out personal care tasks, using your own toiletries, choosing what to wear and how to style your hair and having clean, ironed clothes that fit are all ways of maintaining control and identity. Particular care should be taken in residential settings to ensure that personal laundry is treated with respect and not mixed up or damaged.

The NHS 'Essence of Care' benchmark for personal and oral hygiene[26] focuses on assessment of need, planned care, the care environment and appropriate levels of assistance.

The role of family and carers in supporting the health and wellbeing of people with delirium

Delirium might exist on top of an existing cognitive impairment, or may indeed be a first presenting symptom of dementia. Care plans for carers of people with dementia might incorporate a range of tailored interventions. These may consist of multiple components including:

- individual or group psychological intervention (e.g. CBT)

- peer-support groups with other carers

- support and information by telephone and through the internet

- bespoke training courses

- involvement of *other* family members as well as the primary carer in family meetings.

Those closest to the patient who are not aware of the diagnosis of delirium may feel helpless when faced with unfamiliar, unresolved symptoms and agitation. Health and social care managers should ensure that carers of people with dementia have access to a comprehensive range of respite/short-break services.

It requires effort to make care plans fulfil actual best-practice patient-centred care.

In 1992 Kitwood and Bredin famously shared evidence from studies of different care practices, suggesting that dementia does not *universally* progress in a predictable, linear fashion and that, most importantly, it can vary from person to person.[27] These authors found a need for high-quality interpersonal care that affirms personhood – one that implies recognition, respect and trust. It remains to be seen whether this approach might also apply to delirium.

The importance of the ICU in research

Many studies have focused on physical therapy protocols that use early mobilisation during the ICU stay to prevent neuromuscular dysfunction and progressively advance patients from mechanical ventilation to sitting, standing and eventually walking.

Early progressive mobilisation should be implemented as a top priority in adult ICUs and as an area of clinical focus for ICU physiotherapists.[28] This is a complex intervention that requires careful patient assessment and management, as well as interdisciplinary team collaboration and training.[29]

Endnotes

1   Shields, L., Henderson, V. and Caslake, R. (2017) 'Comprehensive geriatric assessment for prevention of delirium after hip fracture: A systematic review of randomized controlled trials.' *Journal of the American Geriatrics Society* 65, 7, 1559–1565. Accessed on 29/11/2019 at www.ncbi.nlm.nih.gov/pubmed/28407199.

2   See e.g. https://deliriumnetwork.org/wp-content/uploads/2018/05/DRS-R-98.pdf

3   Kenyon-Smith, T., Nguyen, E., Oberai, T. and Jarsma, R. (2019) 'Early mobilization post–hip fracture surgery.' *Geriatric Orthopaedic Surgery and Rehabilitation* 10, 2151459319826431. Accessed on 29/11/2019 at www.ncbi.nlm.nih.gov/pmc/articles/PMC6454638.

4   Drummond, M.J., Dickinson, J.M., Fry, C.S., Walker, D.K. *et al.* (2012) 'Bed rest impairs skeletal muscle amino acid transporter expression, mTORC1 signaling, and protein synthesis in response to essential amino acids in older adults.' *American Journal of Physiology: Endocrinology and Metabolism* 302, 9, E1113–E1133. Accessed on 29/11/2019 at www.ncbi.nlm.nih.gov/pmc/articles/PMC3361979.

5   Lee, S.S., Lo, Y. and Verghese, J. (2019) 'Physical activity and risk of postoperative delirium.' *Journal of the American Geriatrics Society 67*, 11, 2260–2266. Accessed on 29/11/2019 at www.ncbi.nlm.nih.gov/pubmed/31368511.

6   Cortes, O.L., Delgado, S. and Esparza, M. (2019) 'Systematic review and meta-analysis of experimental studies: In-hospital mobilization for patients admitted for medical treatment.' *Journal of Advanced Nursing 75*, 9, 1823–1837. Accessed on 29/11/2019 at www.ncbi.nlm.nih.gov/pubmed/30672011.

7   World Federation of Occupational Therapists (2019) 'About Occupational Therapy.' Accessed on 29/11/2019 at www.wfot.org/about-occupational-therapy.

8   Holly, C. (2019) 'Primary prevention to maintain cognition and prevent acute delirium following orthopaedic surgery.' *Orthopaedic Nursing 38*, 4, 244–250. Accessed on 16/12/2019 at https://journals.lww.com/orthopaedicnursing/Abstract/2019/07000/Primary_Prevention_to_Maintain_Cognition_and.6.aspx.

9   Isaia, G., Astengo, M.A., Tibaldi, V. and Zanocchi, M. (2009) 'Delirium in elderly home-treated patients: A prospective study with 6-month follow-up.' *Age (Dordrecht) 31*, 2, 109–117. Accessed on 29/11/2019 at www.ncbi.nlm.nih.gov/pmc/articles/PMC2693729.

10 van Velthuijsen, E.L., Zwakhalen, S.M.G., Pijpers, E., van de Ven, L.I. *et al.* (2018) 'Effects of a medication review on delirium in older hospitalised patients: A comparative retrospective cohort study.' *Drugs and Aging 35*, 2, 153–161. Accessed on 29/11/2019 at www.ncbi.nlm.nih.gov/pmc/articles/PMC5847150.

11 Health Improvement Scotland (2019) *SIGN 157: Risk Reduction and Management of Delirium. A National Clinical Guideline.* Accessed on 28/11/2019 at www.sign.ac.uk/assets/sign157.pdf.

12 Clegg, A. and Young, J.B. (2011) 'Which medications to avoid in people at risk of delirium: A systematic review.' *Age and Ageing 40*, 1, 23–29. Accessed on 29/11/2019 at www.ncbi.nlm.nih.gov/pubmed/21068014.

13 Victoria State Government (n.d.) 'Preventing and treating incontinence.' Accessed on 29/11/2019 at www2.health.vic.gov.au/hospitals-and-health-services/patient-care/older-people/continence/continence-treating.

14 Alzheimer's Disease International (2014) 'Nutrition and dementia: A review of available research.' Accessed on 29/11/2019 at www.alz.co.uk/sites/default/files/pdfs/nutrition-and-dementia.pdf.

15 Langmore, S.E., Skarupski, K.A., Park, P.S. and Fries, B.E. (2002) 'Predictors of aspiration pneumonia in nursing home residents.' *Dysphagia 17*, 4, 298–307. Accessed on 29/11/2019 at www.ncbi.nlm.nih.gov/pubmed/12355145.

16 Murray, A., Mulkerrin, S. and O'Keeffe, S.T. (2019) 'The perils of "risk feeding".' *Age and Ageing 48*, 4, 478–481. Accessed on 29/11/2019 at https://academic.oup.com/ageing/article-abstract/48/4/478/5423924.

17 Reeve, E., Gnjidic, D., Long, J. and Hilmer, S. (2015) 'A systematic review of the emerging definition of "deprescribing" with network analysis: Implications for future research and clinical practice.' *British Journal of Clinical Pharmacology 80*, 6, 1254–1268. Accessed on 29/11/2019 at www.ncbi.nlm.nih.gov/pubmed/27006985.

18 Growdon, M.E., Shorr, R.I. and Inouye, S.K. (2017) 'The tension between promoting mobility and preventing falls in the hospital.' *JAMA Internal Medicine 177*, 6, 759–760. Accessed on 29/11/2019 at www.ncbi.nlm.nih.gov/pmc/articles/PMC5500203.

19 Growdon, M.E., Shorr, R.I. and Inouye, S.K. (2017) 'The tension between promoting mobility and preventing falls in the hospital.' *JAMA Internal Medicine 177*, 6, 759–760. Accessed on 29/11/2019 at www.ncbi.nlm.nih.gov/pmc/articles/PMC5500203.

20 Babine, R.L., Hyrkäs, K.E., Hallen, S. and Wierman, H.R. (2018) 'Falls and delirium in an acute care setting: A retrospective chart review before and after an organisation-wide interprofessional education.' *Journal of Clinical Nursing 27*, 7–8, e1429–e1441. Accessed on 29/11/2019 at www.ncbi.nlm.nih.gov/pubmed/29314374.

21 Hshieh, T.T., Yang, T., Gartaganis, S.L., Yue, J. and Inouye, S.K. (2018) 'Hospital Elder Life Program: Systematic review and meta-analysis of effectiveness.' *American Journal of Geriatric Psychiatry 26*, 10, 1015–1033. Accessed on 29/11/2019 at www.ncbi.nlm.nih.gov/pubmed/30076080.

22 Gillis, A. and MacDonald, B. (2005) 'Deconditioning in the hospitalized elderly.' *The Canadian Nurse 101*, 6, 16–20. Accessed on 29/11/2019 at www.ncbi.nlm.nih.gov/pubmed/16121472.

23 Kehler, D.S., Theou, O. and Rockwood, K. (2019) 'Bed rest and accelerated aging in relation to the musculoskeletal and cardiovascular systems and frailty biomarkers: A review.' *Experimental Gerontology 126*, 110643. Accessed on 29/11/2019 at www.sciencedirect.com/science/article/pii/S0531556519302062?via%3Dihub.

24 See https://endpjparalysis.org.

25   NHS England (2018) '70 days to end pyjama paralysis.' Accessed on 29/11/2019 at www.england.nhs. uk/2018/03/70-days-to-end-pyjama-paralysis.

26   NHS (2010) 'Essence of Care 2010.' Accessed on 29/11/2019 at https://assets.publishing.service.gov.uk/ government/uploads/system/uploads/attachment_data/file/216691/dh_119978.pdf.

27   Fazio, S., Pace, D., Flinner, J. and Kallmyer, B. (2018) 'The fundamentals of person-centered care for individuals with dementia.' *The Gerontologist 58*, suppl.1, S10–S19. Accessed on 29/11/2019 at https:// academic.oup.com/gerontologist/article/58/suppl_1/S10/4816735#.XXFBSvZqWSk.twitter.

28   Stiller, K. (2013) 'Physiotherapy in intensive care.' *Chest Journal 144*, 3, 825–847. Accessed on 29/11/2019 at https://journal.chestnet.org/article/S0012-3692(13)60598-X/fulltext.

29   Gosselink, R., Bott, J., Johnson, M., Dean, E. *et al.* (2008) 'Physiotherapy for adult patients with critical illness: Recommendations of the European Respiratory Society and European Society of Intensive Care Medicine Task Force on Physiotherapy for Critically Ill Patients.' *Intensive Care Medicine 34*, 7, 1188– 1199. Accessed on 29/11/2019 at https://link.springer.com/article/10.1007%2Fs00134-008-1026-7.

7

Interventions in delirium care

LEARNING OBJECTIVES

Over recent years, enabled and facilitated by evidence-based clinical guidelines, there has been an emerging consensus on the use of non-pharmacological approaches ahead of pharmacological interventions. There is as yet no clear mechanism for the natural history of the diverse presentations of delirium. In this chapter, you will be given an account of possible therapeutic interventions in good delirium care.

I INTRODUCTION
The context

As an overall approach, it is advisable to use interventions that are least restrictive to the patient. But wise interventions are key. Delirium is multifactorial.

The complexity of delirium perhaps implies that a one-size-fits-all pharmacological treatment is unlikely to be of much use. Multicomponent interventions, including non-pharmacological interventions, might be more appropriate for the treatment of delirium, and the outcomes from several such interventions have now been published widely.

The **context** of interventions matters, however, as described by Rycroft-Malone and colleagues:[1]

> Realist synthesis lends itself to the review of complex interventions because it accounts for context as well as outcomes in the process of systematically and transparently synthesising relevant literature. While realist synthesis demands flexible thinking and the ability to deal with complexity, the rewards include the potential for more pragmatic conclusions than alternative approaches to systematic reviewing.

The repertoire of non-pharmacological interventions includes proactive geriatric assessment, multifactorial targeted interventions, staff education and training, and approaches involving family members. The most important actions for clinicians are to identify and correct the underlying causes, and to promote health and wellbeing.

Interventions aimed at reducing high-risk medication use may be a strategy to prevent delirium in hospitalised older adults. The most recent evidence-based guidelines,[2] published in March 2019, recommend the prioritisation of multicomponent, non-pharmacological approaches for the prevention and treatment of delirium.

Approaches to management

A broad overview of a style of approach to management is shown in Box 7.1.

BOX 7.1 BROAD APPROACH

- Coordinate with other members of a multidisciplinary team caring for the patient; ensure and maintain teamwork.
- Assess individual and family psychological and social characteristics.
- Monitor and ensure safety.
- Identify a possible aetiology. The mainstay of treatment is to treat any identifiable underlying cause; note that multiple causes are common.
- At the same time as treating the underlying cause, management should also be directed at the relief of the symptoms of delirium and supportive care until recovery occurs.
- Give attention to acute, life-threatening causes of delirium, including low oxygen, low blood pressure, low glucose and drug intoxication.
- Optimise oxygen saturation when necessary.
- Review medication.
- Provide support and educate the patient and family regarding delirium.
- Follow local antibiotic guidelines where there is evidence of infections and sepsis.
- Ensure good diet, fluid intake and mobility to prevent constipation.
- Initiate interventions for acute conditions; provide other disorder-specific treatment.
- Assess and monitor psychiatric symptoms.
- Correct any biochemical derangements.

- Consider pain as a cause of delirium, but review and reduce pain relief if possible.
- Complete a 'This is me' document (www.alzheimers.org.uk/sites/default/files/migrate/downloads/this_is_me.pdf) and use the information to enhance communication and care for your patient.
- Aim to prevent complications of delirium such as immobility, falls, pressure sores, dehydration, malnourishment and isolation.
- Monitor for any subsequent recovery even if the patient is discharged as a hospital admission.

Environmental and supportive interventions

The patient should be nursed in a good sensory environment, using a reality orientation approach, and with involvement of the multidisciplinary team.

Aspects of a healthy care environment are shown in Box 7.2.

BOX 7.2 A THERAPEUTIC ENVIRONMENT FOR DELIRIUM

- All staff respect the dignity of the patient as a person.
- Lighting levels are appropriate for the time of day.
- Encourage a regular sleep pattern or timetable.
- Establish a quiet relaxing night environment.
- Have a night light in the person's room.
- Use regular and repeated cues to improve personal orientation (examples of orientating cues include clocks, calendars, signs).
- Eliminate unexpected and irritating noise such as television or radio.
- Encourage family to bring in familiar objects and pictures from home and participate in rehabilitation.

Assessments

It can be tempting to over-investigate the patient prior to discharge, when what you are interested in is the level of functioning in a patient's home environment.

Examples of assessments are shown in Box 7.3.

BOX 7.3 ASSESSMENTS

- Encourage safe mobility and provide an appropriate walking aid if necessary. Ask the physiotherapists for help if you are not sure which aid is required.
- Ensure that a 'falls risk assessment' is completed accurately and a 'falls care plan' is in place.
- Ensure that medical staff undertake a comprehensive medication review.
- Consider use of a validated pain assessment tool and ensure pain control.
- Maintain a good intake of food and fluid to avoid constipation. Maintain a clear record through the use of elimination charts.
- If there are problems with continence, undertake a continence assessment.
- Encourage relatives and carers to get involved and to visit regularly.
- Anticipate and avoid complications.

Things to avoid

Some aspects of less good practice are shown in Box 7.4.

BOX 7.4 COMMON FEATURES OF SUBOPTIMAL DELIRIUM CARE

- Catheters
- Cotside bed bars
- Use of restraint, physical or pharmacological – unless absolutely necessary
- Routine use of sedatives
- Arguments with the patient or carer
- Movement of patients around the ward or to other wards
- Constipation
- Use of anticholinergic drugs and other inappropriate drugs

Sleep–wake cycle

Emil Kraepelin, the father of modern psychiatry, in his textbook of psychiatry in 1883, commented on the link between abnormal sleep patterns and poor mental health.[3]

The exact pathophysiology of delirium remains poorly understood, and patients with delirium in the ICU have disturbed sleep–wake cycles, sleep architecture and circadian rhythms. The physiological changes that develop during an episode of delirium further disrupt the individual circadian rhythm, and this could be a vicious cycle for maintaining the delirium.

Melatonin (N-acetyl-5-methoxytryptamine) is a hormone sequentially derived from tryptophan and serotonin and is secreted by the pineal gland during hours of darkness. Melatonin has multiple biological effects, most significantly in the regulation and synchronisation of circadian rhythms. Disturbances in circadian melatonin secretion have been described in a number of patient populations at high risk of delirium. On the basis of this, the abnormal secretion and metabolism of melatonin may play a role in delirium pathogenesis.

In the hypothalamus, orexin plays an important role in awakening. Orexin-containing neurons help integrate metabolism, stress response and circadian rhythms, along with the governance of various neurotransmitters involved in the sleep–wake cycle. It remains unclear whether orexin regulation by suvorexant directly affects the development of delirium.

It is worth noting that sleep and the circadian system exert a strong regulatory influence on immune functions.[4] This is likely to be an important avenue in delirium research. Why we sleep, a fascinating area in itself,[5] might explain an evolutionary advantage to delirium.

II NON-PHARMACOLOGICAL APPROACHES
Psychological and cognitive therapy

Psychological support for patients and relatives is becoming increasingly important in care. Providing reorientation of the person to the world may reduce the development and progress of delirium. There is a wide variety of potential psychological therapies.

Neuro-rehabilitative strategies are mainly based on activities to assist the patient to overcome their psychological trauma and vulnerability and aim to build up the confidence of patients after their critical illness.

Reality orientation

Orientating strategies have been accepted by healthcare staff as helpful in delirium, and clinical care can have a positive effect on psychological wellbeing.

Explaining care and rationalising interventions, making sure that patients are orientated to time and place, and providing patients with information about critical care before admission are all practices that could have a beneficial effect.

Multicomponent interventions

This topic was first introduced in Chapter 3.

The multicomponent intervention should include assessment by a trained and competent healthcare professional, who can recommend actions tailored to the person's needs.

Yale Delirium Prevention Trial

The **Yale Delirium Prevention Trial** evaluated the effectiveness of a multicomponent preventative intervention with patients greater than 70 years of age who were admitted to a general medical floor.[6] The intervention later became the Hospital Elder Life Program (HELP).

Hospital Elder Life Program

The **Hospital Elder Life Program** (HELP), a multicomponent intervention strategy with proven effectiveness and cost-effectiveness in the prevention of delirium and functional decline through targeting of risk factors for delirium, is the most widely disseminated approach. HELP was first developed in 1993. To achieve its goals, the HELP program involves patients, carers and HELP staff members – including an 'Elder Life Specialist', an Elder Life Nurse Specialist, a geriatrician and specially trained volunteers – to work together.[7]

For example, sleep deprivation interventions include minimising and avoiding interruptions, and noise reduction at night, and immobility interventions include early mobilisation, mobility aids and range-of-motion exercise.

ABCDEF bundle

Landmark studies in the prevention of delirium demonstrated the benefit of early mobilisation, leading to better independent function and a shorter duration of mechanical ventilation and delirium.[8] These studies led to the development of the 'ABCDEF bundle' (Assess, prevent and manage pain; Both spontaneous awakening and breathing trials: Choice of analgesia and sedation; Delirium assess, prevent and manage; Early mobility and exercise; Family engagement/empowerment).[9] The ABCDEF bundle focuses on symptom assessment, prevention and management rather than individual disease processes.

The 'TIME bundle'

In Scotland, a comprehensive pathway, incorporating the 'Triggers, Investigate, Manage, Engage' (TIME) bundle,[10] which covers the first two hours of care, and the Scottish Delirium Association (SDA) delirium management pathway provide protocols for good care.

Noise

> **TIP**
> Try to keep the patient's bed away from the ward entrance/exit.

Noise has been *most* studied in the ICU environment with regard to delirium. The ICU is a rapidly changing ward designed to admit severely ill patients. Many studies demonstrate that average hospital and ICU sound levels are excessive and disruptive to patients. Phones ringing and people talking are reported as annoying.

It has been hypothesised that this disturbance of sleep could play an important role in the onset of delirium.[11] Impediments to sleep in the ICU are multifactorial. It is informative to consider ICU sleep disruption within the construct of the Spielman's **3P model** of insomnia or sleep disruption.[12] This model identifies predisposing, precipitating and perpetuating factors. Of these factors, noise (e.g. high sound), light and in-room patient-care activity are modifiable.

The use of earplugs, either alone or with other noise-reducing strategies to promote sleep in ICUs, might be associated with a reduction in incidence of delirium, although this is far from clear.

Light and light therapy

Important risk factors for delirium include older patients, vision impairment, cognitive impairment, severe illness, pre-existing use of antipsychotic medication, sleep deprivation and disturbed sleep–wake rhythm. However, it is now conceded that light is a dominant factor.

> Some questions you could consider about the healthcare environment include:[13]
> - Is there good natural light in bed areas and social spaces?
> - Is the lighting and natural light from windows even (e.g. without pools of light and/or dark areas, stripes or shadows)?

Music

Music interventions in healthcare settings have been shown to promote physical and psychologic health. Music can be delivered in a controlled manner to facilitate movement and positive interactions, and to improve cognition and wellbeing. Altered neurotransmission, which is responsible for causing a calming effect with music, might have various causes.

III PHARMACOLOGICAL INTERVENTIONS
Overview

The main aim of drug treatment may be to treat distressing or dangerous behavioural disturbance (e.g. agitation and hallucinations).

There is now a growing feeling that certain patients with certain features may benefit from certain neurotransmitter interventions, and the way in which we design and interpret pharmacological trials may not encourage such detailed analysis. In the new age of precision medicine, things might change, of course.

Recent theories[14] addressing the pathophysiology of delirium propose that different interacting biological factors disrupt neuronal networks in the brain, resulting in cognitive dysfunction. Delirium prevention has recently been emphasised in national safety reports and as a healthcare quality indicator, and is clearly of significant importance when addressing the care of older adults.

Recent guidelines do *not* recommend pharmacological prevention of delirium first-line, and despite the fact that it is unclear whether pharmacological interventions are effective for the prevention and treatment of delirium in critically ill patients, some of these interventions are currently used routinely in clinical settings. While the exact neurophysiological mechanism and neurological basis of delirium remain sketchy, it has been suggested that imbalances in a number of neurotransmitter pathways lead to the development of delirium.

Imbalances might occur in the release, synthesis and degradation of gamma-aminobutyric acid (GABA), glutamate, acetylcholine, noradrenaline dopamine and serotonin, leading to neurological dysfunction, but how or why they do so are very far from clear currently. Some studies have proposed that these pathways are further influenced by metabolic disturbances often present in critically ill patients such as sepsis, inflammation and ischaemia.

Some manipulations of key neurochemical systems are shown in Box 7.5.

BOX 7.5 NEUROCHEMICAL MANIPULATIONS IN DELIRIUM

Antipsychotics (both typical antipsychotics e.g. haloperidol and atypical antipsychotics e.g. olanzapine, quetiapine, risperidone, aripiprazol, and ziprasidone)

Sedatives (e.g. benzodiazepines)

Dexmedetomidine (an α2-antagonist)

Cholinesterase inhibitors (rivastigmine)

Opioids (e.g. morphine)

Melatonin and melatonin antagonists (e.g. ramelteon)

The current suite of therapeutic agents used for the treatment of delirium have *fundamentally not* developed from an understanding of the underlying neurobiological substrate of delirium, nor any associated complex neurochemical disturbances. Choice of medication is often a balance between uncertain therapeutic benefits versus known adverse effects.

The use of pharmacological agents in delirium have tended to be focused on the treatment of patients with hyperactive delirium at risk of injury to themselves or others.

Recent systematic reviews of drug treatment of delirium have clearly identified the paucity of high-quality randomised controlled trials. A major ethical tenet underlying all clinical research, but in particular randomised clinical trials, has been the concept of clinical equipoise perhaps best classically formulated as 'genuine uncertainty within the expert medical community – not necessarily on the part of the individual investigator – about the preferred treatment'.[15]

It is also the case that drug treatments might address the management (usually by sedation) of patients with 'positive' symptoms, whereas those with 'negative' symptoms remain under-diagnosed and are poorly managed, despite the distress it causes patients.

Future studies should include clinically meaningful measures of patient distress, subsequent memories of delirium, distress, inappropriate continuation of antipsychotic therapy, and long-term outcomes.

Approaches to sedation

Nurses' attitudes toward administering sedative medications to patients receiving mechanical ventilation have evolved recently. In a recent study,[16] more than half of critical care nurses still agree that sedation is necessary to minimise patients' discomfort and distress during mechanical ventilation. Arguably, there is no ideal sedative agent that fulfils the criteria of being inexpensive, rapid in onset and offset, and without local or systemic adverse effects.

Treatment approach with sedation can offer potentially some benefits, including:

- reducing discomfort, anxiety and stress
- facilitating care by providing a calm, cooperative patient who is easy to rouse and capable of communicating pain and other needs.

The use of sedatives and major tranquillisers should be kept to a minimum, however. All sedatives – like many drugs – may cause delirium, especially those with anticholinergic side effects. Many older patients with delirium have hypoactive delirium and arguably do not require yet further sedation. Sedative-hypnotics such as benzodiazepines have even been implicated in the *development* of delirium.[17]

Drug sedation *may* be considered necessary in the following circumstances:

- in order to carry out essential investigations or treatment
- to prevent patients endangering themselves or others
- to relieve distress in a highly agitated patient.

Sedation should only be used in situations as indicated above and should not be used as a form of restraint. If sedatives are prescribed, the prescription should be reviewed regularly and discontinued as soon as possible.

The dopaminergic system and antipsychotics

A recent systematic review of 26 randomised controlled trials and observational studies, evaluating 5607 adult inpatients with delirium, does not support routine use of haloperidol or second-generation antipsychotics for treating delirium in adult inpatients.[18]

The consensus now seems to be that there is a limited therapeutic benefit from antipsychotics in most delirium; therefore, pharmacological interventions should be introduced with great caution to avoid iatrogenic effects, and only if all other non-pharmacological options fail.[19] Therefore, the *routine* use of antipsychotics is not recommended.

The drive to make patients more 'manageable' and less 'distressed' may result in worsened clinical outcomes. These drugs can be considered to be a form of 'chemical restraint', and the concern is that the use of drugs inappropriately in delirium may often be 'treating the providers' rather than serving the best interests of the patient. The National Institute for Health and Care Excellence state that antipsychotic medications for adults should be avoided, especially for those in long-term care or hospitals.[20]

De-escalation techniques should be used for adults who are distressed or pose risk to themselves or others. Should a decision be made to initiate a pharmacological intervention, the NICE guidelines stipulate that first- and second-generation antipsychotics should be used for severe agitation and then only for a short period of time.[21]

Antipsychotics may have appeal as a potential 'quick fix', as compared with non-pharmacological approaches. Powerful incentives in the healthcare system still promote prescription of antipsychotics for patients experiencing delirium, and may have led to the high use of these drugs. Antipsychotics (APs) are a broad class of different drugs and several sub-classes, usually classified as first-generation APs, also known as typical or conventional APs, which include phenothiazines, tioxanthenes, butyrophenones and dibenzoxazepines; second-generation APs; and third-generation APs.

Their inhibiting action on dopamine D_2 receptors are considered the main reason for their use, because of the hypothesis that an excess of dopamine and a deficiency in acetylcholine are involved in the pathophysiology of the syndrome.

SIGN RECOMMENDATION[22]

If commenced, the medication should be reviewed on a daily basis, stopped as soon as the clinical situation allows. Antipsychotics prescribed for delirium should be stopped as soon as the clinical situation allows, typically within 1–2 days. In situations where it is deemed safer to continue antipsychotic therapy for delirium beyond discharge or transfer from hospital, a clear plan for early medication review and follow-up in the community should be agreed.

The use of antipsychotic medications can be associated with neurological side effects, including the development of extrapyramidal side effects, tardive dyskinesia and neuroleptic malignant syndrome. Antipsychotics are associated with greater risk of aspiration pneumonia in hospitals even after extensive adjustment for participant characteristics,[23] which should be considered when prescribing antipsychotics in the hospital.

A NOTE ON HALOPERIDOL

Haloperidol is most frequently used because it has few anticholinergic side effects, few active metabolites and a relatively small likelihood of causing sedation and hypotension. The summary of product characteristics for haloperidol recommends that all patients should have an ECG before and after initiation of haloperidol. Haloperidol causes corrected QT interval – QTc – prolongation, which may lead to *torsade de pointes* and sudden death. The risk of increased QTc elongation is thought to be higher with parental administration and higher doses. The risk and benefit of prescribing haloperidol must be considered in patients who have risk factors for ventricular arrhythmias, and concomitantly prescribing medicines that may also elongate the QTc should be avoided.

The status of haloperidol in the management of delirium is tricky.[24] One study found that the use of haloperidol or ziprasidone, as compared with placebo, in patients with acute respiratory failure or shock and hypoactive or hyperactive delirium in the ICU did not significantly alter the duration of delirium.[25]

Atypical antipsychotics

Recently, some physicians have used the newer antipsychotic medications (risperidone, olanzapine and quetiapine) in the treatment of patients with delirium. Atypical antipsychotics also can have the risk of serious side effects.

Benzodiazepines

Few controlled studies have evaluated the efficacy of benzodiazepines as a monotherapy (i.e. not in combination with other pharmacotherapies) for the treatment of delirium. Except for cases of alcohol and sedative-hypnotic withdrawal where they are the treatment of choice, benzodiazepines are not considered first-line agents in the treatment of delirium-related agitation.

A recent Cochrane review (2020) concluded that there is currently not enough evidence to support the routine use of benzodiazepines for the treatment of cases of delirium excluding those who are cared for in an intensive care unit.[26]

The cholinergic system

Acetylcholine plays an extensive role in attention and consciousness.

Anatomically, cholinergic pathways have widespread interconnections, projecting from the basal forebrain and pontomesencephalon to the striatum and cortex.

A pre-existing cholinergic deficit possibly results in a vulnerability to the cognitive effects of systemic inflammation.

Anticholinergic delirium
Anticholinergic agents are diverse.

The classical anticholinergic clinical syndrome is a manifestation of competitive antagonism of acetylcholine at peripheral and central muscarinic receptors.

Anticholinergic mechanisms may possibly be involved in delirium from hypoxia, hypoglycaemia, thiamine deficiency, traumatic brain injury and stroke.[27]

Drugs with an anticholinergic burden
The concept of anticholinergic burden has been introduced to emphasise the cumulative effect of multiple medications having anticholinergic properties. Deprescribing anticholinergics to reduce state-dependent cognitive impairment or to reduce the risk of delirium in vulnerable demographic and medical populations are reasonable therapeutic rationales.[28]

Drugs in this class are known to affect cognitive function adversely, and could exacerbate or cause dementia symptoms and delirium.

Cholinesterase inhibitors
One systematic review[29] has raised concerns about power of studies already published.

Melatonin
A summary of the current available evidence indicates that there is a complex relationship between melatonin and delirium.

A randomised, placebo-controlled, double-blind trial in 145 elderly internal medicine inpatients reported a reduced risk of delirium in the low-dose (0.5 mg) melatonin-treated group versus placebo.[30] Results of currently available studies on the effect of prophylactic use of melatonin in hospitalised elderly or perioperative patients are controversial.[31]

Dexmedetomidine
Several studies claim that dexmedetomidine may reduce or prevent delirium.

Dexmedetomidine has notably been studied for both prevention of delirium and treatment of delirium-related agitation in ICU patients. Dexmedetomidine has also been shown to reduce the prevalence of delirium following cardiac surgery, to improve early cognition scores in sedated brain-injured and non-brain-injured patients, and to reduce the prevalence of delirium in comparison with benzodiazepines.[32]

Dexmedetomidine is thought to have a number of effects. It:

- exerts its anti-nociceptive effects primarily through alpha-2 receptors in the descending inhibitory nociceptive pathway in the spinal cord

- is a highly selective, centrally acting alpha-2 agonist with sedative, analgesic and anxiolytic properties

- decreases arousal

- decreases sympathetic activity

- acts as an agonist in the locus coeruleus and inhibits noradrenaline release, haemodynamic and neuroendocrinal stress responses (including of cortisol), resulting in decreased heart rate and blood pressure

- is also thought to have mild cholinergic activity which may favourably affect the sleep–wake cycle.

Dexmedetomidine should be administered with caution to certain patients. The drug product monograph indicates an increased risk of adverse effects with abrupt discontinuation.[33]

Two published meta-analyses suggested that dexmedetomidine might decrease the occurrence of post-operative delirium, compared with other active sedative drugs, in adult patients who underwent cardiac surgery; and the main conclusion of a recent review was that elderly patients who underwent noncardiac surgery and received dexmedetomidine intervention had a significantly lower occurrence of post-operative delirium than those who received placebo.[34]

Long QT syndrome

The FDA issued 'black box' warnings in April 2005 and June 2008 regarding the use of antipsychotic agents in the elderly.

The QT prolonging effects of antipsychotic and other agents are described in the British National Formulary.[35] QTP is the best predictor of *torsade de pointes*, a malignant ventricular dysrhythmia.

Endnotes

1   Rycroft-Malone, J., McCormack, B., Hutchinson, A.M., DeCorby, K. *et al.* (2012) 'Realist synthesis: Illustrating the method for implementation research.' *Implementation Science 7*, 33. Accessed on 29/11/2019 at https://implementationscience.biomedcentral.com/articles/10.1186/1748-5908-7-33.

2   Health Improvement Scotland (2019) *SIGN 157: Risk Reduction and Management of Delirium. A National Clinical Guideline.* Accessed on 28/11/2019 at www.sign.ac.uk/assets/sign157.pdf.

3   Cited in Lockley, S.W. and Foster, R.G. (2012) *Sleep: A Very Short Introduction.* Oxford: Oxford University Press, p.97.

4   Besedovsky, L., Lange, T. and Born, J. (2012) 'Sleep and immune function.' *Pflugers Archiv: European Journal of Physiology 483*, 1, 121–137. Accessed on 29/11/2019 at www.ncbi.nlm.nih.gov/pmc/articles/PMC3256323.

5   Walker, M. (2017) *Why We Sleep.* London: Penguin Random House.

6   Inouye, S.K., Bogardus, S.T. Jr, Charpentier, P.A., Leo-Summers, L. *et al.* (1999) 'A multi-component intervention to prevent delirium in hospitalized older patients.' *New England Journal of Medicine 340*, 9, 669–676. Accessed on 29/11/2019 at www.ncbi.nlm.nih.gov/pubmed/10053175.

7   Hospital Elder Life Program (HELP) for Prevention of Delirium: https://hospitalelderlifeprogram.org.

8   Schweickert, W.D., Pohlman, M.C., Pohlman, A.S., Nigos, C. *et al.* (2009) 'Early physical and occupational therapy in mechanically ventilated, critically ill patients: A randomised controlled trial.' *Lancet 373*, 1874–1882.

9   Marra, A., Ely, E.W., Pandharipande, P.P. and Patel, M.B. (2017) 'The ABCDEF bundle in critical care.' *Critical Care Clinics 33*, 2, 225–243. Accessed on 29/11/2019 at www.ncbi.nlm.nih.gov/pmc/articles/PMC5351776.

10   Bauernfreund, Y., Butler, M., Ragavan, S. and Sampson, E.L. (2018) 'TIME to think about delirium: Improving detection and management on the acute medical unit.' *BMJ Open Quality 7*, e000200. Accessed on 29/11/2019 at https://bmjopenquality.bmj.com/content/7/3/e000200#DC2.

11   Watson, P.L., Ceriana, P. and Fanfulla, F. (2013) 'Delirium: Is sleep important?' *Best Practice and Research Clinical Anaesthesiology 26*, 3, 355–366. Accessed on 29/11/2019 at www.ncbi.nlm.nih.gov/pmc/articles/PMC3808245.

12   Perlis, M., Shaw, P., Cano, G. and Espie, C. (n.d.) 'Models of Insomnia.' Accessed on 29/11/2019 at www.med.upenn.edu/cbti/assets/user-content/documents/ppsmmodelsofinsomnia2011 5theditionproof.pdf.

13   It is worth consulting a resource such 'Is your ward dementia friendly? The EHE Environmental Assessment Tool' from the King's Fund: www.kingsfund.org.uk/sites/default/files/EHE-dementia-assessment-tool.pdf.

14   See e.g. Maldonado, J.R. (2018) 'Delirium pathophysiology: An updated hypothesis of the etiology of acute brain failure.' *International Journal of Geriatric Psychiatry 33*, 11, 1428–1457. Accessed on 16/12/2019 at www.ncbi.nlm.nih.gov/pubmed/29278283.

15   Doig, C.J., Page, S.A., McKee, J.L., Moore, E.E. *et al.* (2019) 'Ethical considerations in conducting surgical research in severe complicated intra-abdominal sepsis.' *World Journal of Emergency Surgery 14*, 39. Accessed on 28/11/2019 at https://wjes.biomedcentral.com/articles/10.1186/s13017-019-0259-9.

16   Guttormson, J.L., Chian, L., Tracy, M.F., Hetland, B. and Mandrekar, J. (2019) 'Nurses' attitudes and practices related to sedation: A national survey.' *American Journal of Critical Care 28*, 4, 255–263. Accessed on 29/11/2019 at www.ncbi.nlm.nih.gov/pubmed/31263007.

17   Alagiakrishnan, K. and Wiens, C.A. (2004) 'An approach to drug induced delirium in the elderly.' *Postgraduate Medical Journal 80*, 388–393. Accessed on 29/11/2019 at https://pmj.bmj.com/content/80/945/388.

18   Nikooie, R., Neufeld, K.J., Oh, E.S., Wilson, L.M. *et al.* (2019) 'Antipsychotics for treating delirium in hospitalized adults: A systematic review.' *Annals of Internal Medicine 171*, 7, 485–495. Accessed on 29/11/2019 at https://annals.org/aim/fullarticle/2749495/antipsychotics-treating-delirium-hospitalized-adults-systematic-review.

19   van Wissen, K. and Blanchard, D. (2019) 'Anti-psychotics for treatment of delirium in hospitalized non-ICU patients: A Cochrane Review Summary.' *International Journal of Nursing Practice 25*, 4, e12741. Accessed on 29/11/2019 at https://onlinelibrary.wiley.com/doi/abs/10.1111/ijn.12741.

20   National Institute for Healthcare and Excellence (NICE) (2014) 'Delirium in adults: Quality standard.' Accessed on 29/11/2019 at www.nice.org.uk/guidance/qs63/resources/delirium-in-adults-pdf-2098785962437.

21   National Institute for Healthcare and Excellence (NICE) (2014) 'Delirium in adults: Quality statement 3: Use of antipsychotic medication for people who are distressed.' Accessed on 29/11/2019 at www.nice. org.uk/guidance/qs63/chapter/Quality-statement-3-Use-of-antipsychotic-medication-for-people-who-are-distressed.

22   Health Improvement Scotland (2019) *SIGN 157: Risk Reduction and Management of Delirium. A National Clinical Guideline.* Accessed on 28/11/2019 at www.sign.ac.uk/assets/sign157.pdf.

23   Herzig, S.J., LaSalvia, M.T., Naidus, E., Rothberg, M.B. *et al.* (2017) 'Antipsychotics and the risk of aspiration pneumonia in individuals hospitalized for nonpsychiatric conditions: A cohort study.' *Journal of the American Geriatrics Society 65*, 12, 2580–2586. Accessed on 29/11/2019 at www.ncbi.nlm.nih.gov/pubmed/29095482.

24   Neufeld, K.J., Needham, D.M., Oh, E.S., Wilson, L.M. *et al.* (2019) 'Antipsychotics for the prevention and treatment of delirium.' *Comparative Effectiveness Review 219.* Accessed on 29/11/2019 at www.ncbi.nlm. nih.gov/pubmed/31509366.

25   Girard, T.D., Exline, M.C., Carson, S.S., Hough, C.L. *et al.* (2018) 'Haloperidol and ziprasidone for treatment of delirium in critical illness.' *New England Journal of Medicine 379*, 26, 2506–2516. Accessed on 29/11/2019 at www.ncbi.nlm.nih.gov/pubmed/30346242.

26   Li, Y., Ma, J., Jin, Y., Li, N. *et al.* (2020) 'Benzodiazepines for treatment of patients with delirium excluding those who are cared for in an intensive care unit.' *Cochrane Database of Systematic Reviews, 2.* Accessed on 11/03/2020 at https://www.cochranelibrary.com/cdsr/doi/10.1002/14651858.CD012670.pub2/pdf/full.

27   Hshieh, T.T., Fong, T.G., Marcantonio, E.R. and Inouye, S.K. (2008) 'Cholinergic deficiency hypothesis in delirium: A synthesis of current evidence.' *Journals of Gerontology. Series A, Biological Sciences and Medical Sciences 63*, 7, 764–772. Accessed on 29/11/2019 at www.ncbi.nlm.nih.gov/pmc/articles/PMC2917793.

28   Andrade, C. (2019) 'Anticholinergic drug exposure and the risk of dementia: There is modest evidence for an association but not for causality.' *Journal of Clinical Psychiatry 80*, 4. Accessed on 29/11/2019 at www.ncbi.nlm.nih.gov/pubmed/31390497.

29   Tampi, R.R., Tampi, D.J. and Ghori, A.K. (2016) 'Acetylcholinesterase inhibitors for delirium on older adults.' *American Journal of Alzheimer's Disease and Other Dementias 31*, 4, 305–310. Accessed on 29/11/2019 at www.ncbi.nlm.nih.gov/pubmed/26646113.

30   Al-Aama, T., Brymer, C., Gutmanis, I., Woolmore-Goodwin, S.M., Esbaugh, J. and Dasgupta, M. (2011) 'Melatonin decreases delirium in elderly patients: A randomized, placebo-controlled trial.' *International Journal of Geriatric Psychiatry 26*, 7, 687–694. Accessed on 29/11/2019 at www.ncbi.nlm.nih.gov/pubmed/20845391.

31   Zhang, Q., Gao, F., Zhang, S., Sun, W. and Li, Z. (2019) 'Prophylactic use of exogenous melatonin and melatonin receptor agonists to improve sleep and delirium in the intensive care units: A systematic review and meta-analysis of randomized controlled trials.' *Sleep and Breathing 23*, 4, 1059–1070. Accessed on 29/11/2019 at www.ncbi.nlm.nih.gov/pubmed/31119597.

32   Clancy, O., Edginton, T., Casarin, A. and Vizcaychipi, M.P., (2015) 'The psychological and neurocognitive consequences of critical illness: A pragmatic review of current evidence.' *Journal of the Intensive Care Society 16*, 3, 226–233. Accessed on 29/11/2019 at www.ncbi.nlm.nih.gov/pmc/articles/PMC5606436.

33   Ungarian, J., Rankin, J.A. and Then, K.L. (2019) 'Delirium in the intensive care unit: Is dexmedetomidine effective?' *Critical Care Nurse 39*, 4, e8–e21. Accessed on 29/11/2019 at www.ncbi.nlm.nih.gov/pubmed/31371374.

34   Zeng, H., Li, Z., He, J. and Fu, W. (2019) 'Dexmedetomidine for the prevention of postoperative delirium in elderly patients undergoing noncardiac surgery: A meta-analysis of randomized controlled trials.' *PLOS One.* Accessed on 29/11/2019 at https://journals.plos.org/plosone/article?id=10.1371/journal.pone.0218088.

35   See e.g. National Institute for Health and Care Excellence (2019) 'Psychosis and related disorders: Advice of Royal College of Psychiatrists on doses of antipsychotic drugs above BNF upper limit.' Accessed on 16/12/2019 at https://bnf.nice.org.uk/treatment-summary/psychoses-and-related-disorders.html.

8

Outcomes after an episode of delirium

LEARNING OBJECTIVES
The idea that delirium presents no inherent risk and is completely reversible is looking increasingly untenable. Often clinicians will be asked what to expect after the person has made an initial recovery from the current delirium episode. This chapter considers some of the possible themes of that discussion.

Introduction

It is important to recognise that the prevalence, causes, treatment and outcomes associated with delirium may vary substantially depending on where any patient is along any particular disease trajectory.

Patients experiencing delirium with failure to recover fully after discharge from hospital might be especially vulnerable to subsequent adverse events.[1]

Further studies will improve organisational understanding of clinical outcomes for acute patients experiencing delirium across the whole system. This will in turn facilitate quality improvement initiatives to improve patient care and modernisation of community service (see Chapter 12).

Pressure on acute hospitals

Acute hospitals are themselves under considerable pressure to shorten length of stays and avoid delays associated with complex discharges. Specialist models of inpatient care, such as receiving comprehensive geriatric assessment, have been shown to reduce the risk of adverse outcomes.

Adaptation of the physical environment to promote wellbeing

Rehabilitation, reablement and intermediate care all stem from a desire to enable individuals to live independent lives with meaning and purpose, to empower individuals to be self-determined, and to avoid dependency on health and social care.

Therapy is so important. The primary goal of occupational therapy is:

> to enable people to participate in the activities of everyday life. Occupational therapists achieve this outcome by working with people and communities to enhance their ability to engage in the occupations they want to, need to, or are expected to do, or by modifying the occupation or the environment to better support their occupational engagement.[2]

Technology that assists people with long-term health conditions, and who are at risk of frequent hospital admissions as a result, has proved to be desirable.

There is good evidence regarding the better use of healthcare resources after occupational therapy programmes carried out in the community. Here, a reduction in readmission rates, treatment services on discharge and risks at home have been reported, in addition to an improvement in quality of life for the patient and their carer or family.[3]

Care planning

In theory, planning for the future by a person at a stage when they have mental capacity to make decisions about the future arguably is more empowering than surrogate decision-making. In addition to impaired communication of the decision itself, a patient's ability to make medical decisions is often diminished or lacking, depending on the severity of the delirium and the complexity of the specific decisions to be made. In the last weeks of life, many complex decisions – related to factors such as discharge planning, treatment discontinuation or even death – need to be addressed.

Because patients with delirium often have compromised capacity and autonomy, surrogate decision-makers must make many of these decisions. In order to avoid unnecessary hospital admissions and empower people with regard to their own health and wellbeing, people with long-term conditions are encouraged to have a care and support plan that can anticipate needs for optimal wellbeing, as well as promoting strengths and capabilities and anticipating any deterioration. Such plans will include signposting to both NHS, social care, voluntary or community organisations for support. Carers need to be informed of their right to have a new or updated adult carer support plan, and support needs to be in place before the patient is discharged to their home.

'**Personalised care and support planning**', currently adopted in policy by NHS England,[4] is a series of 'facilitated conversations' in which the person – or those who know them well, including unpaid family carers – can actively participate to explore options for the future. It is intended that such an approach results in the outcomes and solutions developed having real meaning to the person. The personalised care and support plan should be developed following an initial holistic assessment of the person's health and wellbeing needs. The person, or those closest to them, work with their health and social care professionals to complete this assessment which then leads to producing an agreed personalised care and support plan.

Advance care planning for an adult who will receive palliative care should include documentation of the patient's understanding of diagnosis, prognosis and expectations, as well as decisions about end-of-life care and death. Further issues are discussed in Chapter 11.

The role of family and carers in enabling people with delirium to live well

Unpaid family carers play a significant role in enabling people with health and social care needs to remain independent and at home. It is important that carers are supported to look after their own health and wellbeing, and to access support to enable them to continue with their caring role, including financial resources such as carers' allowance or carers' benefit. It is important to ensure that carers can access correct, accurate and up-to-date information, advice and support relevant to their caring identity.

Possible outcomes after post-operative delirium

Education concerning the risk factors and the major clinical manifestations underlies post-operative delirium prevention and principles and practice of its treatment.[5] Post-operative delirium is a special entity which deserves a special mention. Prospective studies and trials are needed to address the relationships between pre-operative cognitive impairment and patient outcomes to inform and identify best practices.[6]

In patients undergoing a noncardiac operation and in patients admitted to intensive care units, delirium might be associated with a number of outcomes:[7]

- increased rate of probability of death

- cognitive decline

- readmission to hospital

- increased hospital length of stay

- greater likelihood of being transferred to a residential setting

- decreased health-related quality of life

- a decline in activities of daily living.

It is possible that delirium ultimately sets off a cascade of events, starting with failure of the integrity of the blood barrier, neuroinflammation, stress response and alterations in neurotransmission.[8] A bi-phasic pattern of cognitive decline after delirium has been hypothesised.[9] The acute decline represents the impact of transient precipitating events, such as anaesthesia, surgery and hospitalisation, which resolve relatively early. The later effects, however, suggest a more long-lasting process

Overview of outcomes following a delirium episode

Examples of common outcomes from delirium include:

- 'patient experience' (a focus of Chapter 9)

- falls

- a longer hospital stay

- subsyndromal delirium

- cognitive impairment

- neuropsychiatric symptoms

- transfer to care home

- 'disablement'

- transfer back home

- 'post-ICU syndrome'

- readmissions

- mortality.

A universal definition of **'recovery'** from delirium is lacking.[10] A distinction might be made between symptomatic and overall recovery, as well as between long- and short-term outcomes. Cognitive recovery could be central to defining recovery in delirium, which is interesting in itself as the initial behavioural changes can be striking.

Although most delirium is short-lived, longer-term effects of an episode of delirium may impact a patient's ability to recover from surgery and hospitalisation, and this matters because these consequences can be difficult to manage in all care settings following an episode.

Delirium and falls

There has historically been a drive towards preventing persons experiencing delirium from mobilising in case they experience falls. This drive is especially intense in risk-averse cultures.

Preventing delirium might prevent falls.[11]

In 2015, Hshieh and colleagues[12] found that delirium incidence decreased as a result of reported interventions with a corresponding reduction in the fall rate.

Delirium and the increased length of stay in hospitals

Acute illness accompanied by delirium is generally associated with longer hospital stays. Several explanations have been proposed. For example, a greater severity of illness might result in both more frequent delirium and longer hospital stays, independently of each other.

Subsyndromal delirium

Subsyndromal delirium (SSD) can happen at any time.

SSD in patients is associated with outcomes midway between patients not experiencing delirium and those with definite full syndromal delirium (FSD). The recognition of SSD is hampered by the issue that many patients experiencing delirium have mild non-specific symptoms that could be misattributed to subsyndromal delirium (e.g. mild inattention, sleep difficulties, agitation, drug-induced sedation).

Emergency admission of an older patient presenting with FSD or SSD might be a strong potential indicator of risk of death; there is perhaps a 'dose-response relationship' between mortality and delirium, FSD having the greatest risk and SSD having intermediate risk.[13]

Subsequent cognitive impairment

If there are concerns about cognitive impairment developing in the following months, advise the patient/carers to see their general practitioner.

Lipowski classically stated that **delirium may increase the risk of dementia**.[14] There is some evidence that patients who develop post-operative delirium represent a subgroup at risk for prolonged and even permanent cognitive disorder that may negatively affect health-related quality of life.[15]

A prospective cohort study identified delirium as an independent predictor of long-term cognitive impairment among medical ICU patients attempting to recover from critical illness requiring mechanical ventilation.[16] Alternatively, delirium may be associated with a pre-existing higher rate of cognitive decline that was not detected at baseline. Delirium may serve as a robust marker for persons with poor cognitive reserve *at heightened risk* for accelerated long-term cognitive decline.

Neuropsychiatric symptoms

Mental health disorders associated with an ICU stay include anxiety, apathy, compulsions, impulsivity, depression, post-traumatic stress disorder (PTSD) and complicated grief reactions and bereavement for families. Acute stress specifically comprises experiences that are common for patients in critical care units: fear of dying, invasive treatments, pain and discomfort, inability to communicate and hallucinatory delusions.[17]

It is possible that impaired recall of the ICU episode, as well as interfering hallucinations or delusions, contributes to the post-traumatic stress. A recent systematic review[18] of PTSD in general ICU survivors demonstrated that the prevalence of substantial post-ICU PTSD symptoms is high, and symptoms persist over time; this review also revealed that post-ICU PTSD may have a substantial impact on quality of life.[19] Studies have focused on prevalence of PTSD in survivors of different ICUs at three months to one year post discharge, and have reported a varying prevalence ranging from 9% to 30%.

The use of an 'ICU diary' given to the patient who has experienced delirium at discharge might offer some benefit. By providing objective information to patients, ICU diaries can allow survivors to make sense of their distressing experience and become reorientated to reality.

Transfer to a care home

Current health and social care policy in the UK promotes 'independent living', and a key outcome after hospital admission is the maintenance of independence. Discharge decisions, particularly the delays which can be associated with transfers to care homes, may be affected by the presence of delirium. Admission to a care home is inevitably a significant life-changing event for the individual and their family. Decisions made as hospital inpatients may be prompted by a crisis, and important external factors, such as finances and availability of home care, influence individual outcome.

There is a formidable body of international research which explores care-home admission in people with a long-term cognitive impairment living in the community. By comparison, the experiences of older adults admitted to a care home following hospital admission lack much rigorous research.

Decisions about care-home admission are recognised to be difficult for everyone, as they tend to be somewhat 'ad hoc' and attempt to balance competing individual health and social needs with those of carers. Healthcare professionals have a key role in supporting decision-making, but this again needs calm communication between healthcare professionals, patients and carers.

New care-home admission can be necessary to address care needs which cannot be met in the community, but it is a significant and life-changing event which many older people fear and do not completely plan for. Care-home admission from hospital is common, although rates vary significantly between hospitals, and may happen somewhat prematurely in people who have experienced an episode of delirium due to the emotional 'shock' of delirium. Returning to and remaining at home after acute hospital care is therefore a highly desirable outcome for patients, health services and society.

'Disablement'

The literature on disability, in particular how people go from independence to dependence through disability, is not straightforward. The disabling process can be conceptualised as a series of transitions between states of disability and independence.[20] As the population ages, disability is becoming an increasingly important public health problem.

Recent evidence has suggested that disability is actually a 'dynamic process' with numerous considerations.[21] While the likelihood of recovery from a single episode of disability is very high, older persons who have recovered independent function are at high risk of recurrent disability.

A 2004 study reported by Hardy and Gill[22] proposed that newly disabled older persons recover independent ADL function at rates far exceeding those previously thought, but that recovery from disability is often short-lived. The significance of this is that additional efforts are warranted to maintain independence in this high-risk group.

Transfer back home

Any family/carers will to a large degree have to take responsibility if a patient with delirium is discharged back home. It is therefore necessary to liaise with the family/carers regarding timely discharge arrangements, and to ensure that the care package, including assistive equipment, is appropriate for the function anticipated at discharge. It is also important to discuss with family/carers whether they need extra support, as 'burn-out' and 'carer stress' are very real phenomena and might lead to readmission.

The stress of a hospital admission for delirium, for both patients and carers, should never be underestimated. It is a goal that people are in hospital for the shortest possible time, ensuring that medical and nursing needs that can only be delivered in an acute hospital setting happen there, such as identifying and managing a relevant acute medical problem. However, many patients with delirium are obliged to undertake prolonged assessments while delirious and in a hospital environment. This is a time-consuming process, potentially lowering the morale of patients who feel they are being examined in a 'pass/fail' way, and all this time spent contributes to the deconditioning.

A definition of '**Discharge to Assess**'[23] is:

> Where people who are clinically optimised and do not require an acute hospital bed, but may still require care services are provided with short term, funded support to be discharged to their own home (where appropriate) or another community setting. Assessment for longer-term care and support needs is then undertaken in the most appropriate setting and at the right time for the person.

Using a combination of 'Home First'[24] and 'Discharge to Assess' approaches, patients are supported to return home to recover from their admission to hospital. Aspects of this successful approach include:

- Put people and their families at the centre of decisions.

- Take steps to understand both the perspectives of the patient and their carers and the communities they live in.

- Provide simple access to information, advice and services.

- Make decisions on long-term care needs after individuals have had a period of recovery and rehabilitation.

- Develop an awareness of services actually available at home.[25]

It is worth noting that physiotherapy is believed to be relatively cost-effective and delivers value within available resources. As well as achieving admission or readmission avoidance and the delay or prevention of the need for complex or residential care, physiotherapists use **an asset-based approach** within a community environment to support a long-term focus on health and wellbeing – in other words, drawing on the strengths and capabilities of patients. Physiotherapists also ensure the best use of resources to deliver a personal care plan funded by a direct payment. The use of physical or medical restraints that impede mobility are also recognised risk factors for delirium. Other barriers to mobility include bed rest orders, unclear physician orders regarding mobility, inadequate referral for physiotherapy assessment and support, limited nursing time, and concerns about potential falls risks. The implications for human rights are discussed further in Chapter 10.

Post-ICU syndrome

Neuroinflammation can be precipitated by systemic inflammatory insults such as infection or sepsis, with increased production of cytokines and reactive oxygen species activating microglia and leading to disruption of core networks in the brain. The relationship between delirium and inflammation is important, because protracted neuroinflammation could lead to long-term deterioration following the episode of delirium.

For example:[26]

There is also robust evidence that these inflammatory insults have a deleterious effect on the consolidation of new memories in contextual fear-conditioning experiments but these studies do not explain why relatively banal infections such as urinary tract infections in the elderly population produce the profound cognitive changes observed during episodes of delirium but have limited effects in younger, healthy populations.

Inflammation is common in very many illnesses seen in the ICU. Regular physical activity, even at a low intensity, might reduce the pro-inflammatory profile of acute and chronic disease, and the evidence is being confirmed across a number of different approaches.[27] It is possible that abnormal levels of inflammatory biomarkers are associated with loss of muscle mass and strength and delirium onset perhaps through enhanced oxidative stress mechanisms.[28]

Poor mobilising during hospitalisation has been recognised as a risk for **hospital-related functional decline**. An updated systematic review into physiotherapy in intensive care concluded with the suggestion that early and progressive mobilisation should be implemented as a matter of priority in all adult ICUs and as an area of clinical focus for ICU physiotherapists.[29]

The term 'post-intensive care syndrome' has been developed to describe a diverse range of physical, cognitive or psychological symptoms that persist in critically ill patients or their family members subsequent to an ICU stay.

Readmissions

Readmissions can be sign of poor continuity of care between primary care and secondary care, which is so important in delirium care at a systems level; reasons include poor communication between hospital staff and staff in the community, poor care and support planning and the failure to identify a 'named person' responsible for care.[30]

In a recent study[31] of patients in a community hospital in Northern California, a significant association between inpatient delirium and risk of hospital readmission within 30 days of discharge was found. The results cumulatively suggest that patients with delirium are particularly vulnerable in the period following hospitalisation.

Strategies to reduce readmissions for patients who have had to experience delirium in hospital might in future need to focus on prevention of hospital-acquired delirium. There is a strong case for adequate carer and patient education and support after discharge. Readmissions, rather inevitably, can also put the health and wellbeing of a person recovering from delirium at risk. The structural discontinuities in care are significant, but might be mitigated against by an ethos more geared more toward patients' needs rather than the operational processes of health providers or the demands of specific diseases.[32]

Mortality

It is quite possible that patients with delirium are on average more severely ill from precipitating factors.

A 2017 study by Inouye and colleagues found a fourfold increased risk of death at 90 days following hospitalisation, with restraining devices and 'noxious insults' as possible contributing factors.[33]

Delirium has been shown to be an independent marker for increased mortality among older hospital patients at 12 months post-hospital admission.[34] Relevant to the 'aberrant stress response' view of delirium, studies have shown that mammals can directly die from prolonged exposure to stress, with gastric ulceration and neurotoxicity as proven pathologies post-mortem.[35]

In one study, it was found that one in three acutely ill hospitalised older adults who suffered hypoactive or mixed delirium died *in* the hospital.[36] This finding on the high frequency and poor prognosis associated with hypoactive delirium has particular relevance for clinical practice, since it is documented that physicians and nurses have greater difficulty in identifying hypoactive delirium in the first place.

In a recent systematic review and meta-analysis,[37] a reduced level of arousal on admission to hospital with general medical illnesses was found to be associated with a substantial increased risk of in-hospital mortality. Patients with reduced level of arousal should therefore be identified as having a high risk of in-hospital death, and their care should be more of a priority than it sometimes is.

Endnotes

1   Cole, M.G., McCusker, J., Bailey, R., Bonnycastle, M. *et al.* (2017) 'Partial and no recovery from delirium after hospital discharge predict increased adverse effects.' *Age and Ageing 46*, 1, 90–95. Accessed on 29/11/2019 at https://academic.oup.com/ageing/article/46/1/90/2605678.

2   World Federation of Occupational Therapists (2019) 'About Occupational Therapy.' Accessed on 29/11/2019 at www.wfot.org/about-occupational-therapy.

3   Cuevas-Lara, C., Izquierdo, M., Gutiérrez-Valencia, M., Marin-Epelde, I. *et al.* (2019) 'Effectiveness of occupational therapy interventions in acute geriatric wards: A systematic review.' *Maturitas 127*, 43–50. Accessed on 29/11/2019 at www.ncbi.nlm.nih.gov/pubmed/31351519.

4   NHS England (n.d.) 'Personalised care and support planning.' Accessed on 29/11/2019 at www.england. nhs.uk/ourwork/patient-participation/patient-centred/planning.

5   Kyziridis, T.C. (2006) 'Post-operative delirium after hip fracture treatment – a review of the current literature.' *GMS Psycho-Social-Medicine 3*, 1. Accessed on 29/11/2019 at www.ncbi.nlm.nih.gov/pmc/articles/PMC2736510.

6   Mahanna-Gabrielli, E., Schenning, K.J., Eriksson, L.I., Browndyke, J.N. *et al.* (2019) 'State of the clinical science of perioperative brain health: Report from the American Society of Anesthesiologists Brain Health Initiative Summit 2018.' *British Journal of Anaesthesia 123*, 4, 464–478. Accessed on 29/11/2019 at www.sciencedirect.com/science/article/pii/S0007091219305562.

7   Crocker, E., Beggs, T., Hassan, A., Denault, A. *et al.* (2016) 'Long-term effects of postoperative delirium in patients undergoing cardiac operation: A systematic review.' *Annals of Thoracic Surgery 102*, 4, 1391–1399. Accessed on 29/11/2019 at www.ncbi.nlm.nih.gov/pubmed/27344279.

8   Inouye, S.K., Marcantonio, E.R., Kosar, C.M., Tommet, D. *et al.* (2016) 'The short- and long-term relationship between delirium and cognitive trajectory in older surgical patients.' *Alzheimer's and Dementia 12*, 7, 766–775. Accessed on 29/11/2019 at www.ncbi.nlm.nih.gov/pmc/articles/PMC4947419.

9   Inouye, S.K., Marcantonio, E.R., Kosar, C.M., Tommet, D. *et al.* (2016) 'The short- and long-term relationship between delirium and cognitive trajectory in older surgical patients.' *Alzheimer's and Dementia 12*, 7, 766–775. Accessed on 29/11/2019 at www.ncbi.nlm.nih.gov/pmc/articles/PMC4947419

10   Adamis, D., Devaney, A., Shanahan, E., McCarthy, G. and Meagher, D., (2015) 'Defining "recovery" for delirium research: A systematic review.' *Age and Ageing 44*, 2, 318–321. Accessed on 29/11/2019 at www.ncbi.nlm.nih.gov/pubmed/25476590.

11   Babine, R., Farrington, S. and Wierman, H.R. (2013) 'HELP© prevent falls by preventing delirium.' *Nursing 43*, 5, 18–21. Accessed on 29/11/2019 at https://journals.lww.com/nursing/Fulltext/2013/05000/HELP__prevent_falls_by_preventing_delirium.7.aspx.

12   Hshieh, T.T., Yue, J., Oh, E., Puelle, M. et al. (2015) 'Effectiveness of multicomponent nonpharmacological delirium interventions, a meta-analysis.' JAMA Internal Medicine 175, 4, 512–520. Accessed on 29/11/2019 at www.ncbi.nlm.nih.gov/pmc/articles/PMC4388802.

13   Diwell, R.A., Davis, D.H., Vickerstaff, V. and Sampson, E.L. (2018) 'Key components of the delirium syndrome and mortality: Greater impact of acute change and disorganised thinking in a prospective cohort study.' BMC Geriatrics 18, 24. Accessed on 29/11/2019 at www.ncbi.nlm.nih.gov/pmc/articles/PMC5785815.

14   Lipowski, Z.J. (1990) Delirium: Acute Confusional States. New York, NY: Oxford University Press.

15   Antunes, M., Norton, V., Moreira, J.F., Moreira, A. and Abelha, F. (2013) 'Quality of life in patients with postoperative delirium.' European Journal of Anaesthesiology 30, 11. Accessed on 29/11/2019 at https://journals.lww.com/ejanaesthesiology/Fulltext/2013/06001/Quality_of_life_in_patients_with_post-operative.33.aspx.

16   Girard, T.D., Jackson, J.C., Pandharipande, P.P., Pun, B.T. et al. (2010) 'Delirium as a predictor of long-term cognitive impairment in survivors of critical illness.' Critical Care Medicine 38, 7, 1513–1520. Accessed on 29/11/2019 at www.ncbi.nlm.nih.gov/pmc/articles/PMC3638813.

17   Mouncey, P.R., Wade, D., Richards-Belle, A. et al. (2019) 'A nurse-led, preventive, psychological intervention to reduce PTSD symptom severity in critically ill patients: The POPPI feasibility study and cluster RCT.' Health Services and Delivery Research 730. Accessed on 29/11/2019 at www.ncbi.nlm.nih.gov/books/NBK545672.

18   Davydow, D.S., Gifford, J.M., Desai, S.V., Needham, D.M. and Bienvenu, O.J. (2008) 'Posttraumatic stress disorder in general intensive care unit survivors: A systematic review.' General Hospital Psychiatry 30, 5, 412–434. Accessed on 29/11/2019 at www.ncbi.nlm.nih.gov/pmc/articles/PMC2572638.

19   Grover, S., Sahoo, S., Chakrabarti, S. and Avasthi, A. (2019) 'Post-traumatic stress disorder (PTSD) related symptoms following an experience of delirium.' Journal of Psychosomatic Research 123, 109725. Accessed on 29/11/2019 at www.ncbi.nlm.nih.gov/pubmed/31376870.

20   Hardy, S.E., Dubin, J.A., Holford, T.R. and Gill, T.M. (2005) 'Transitions between states of disability and independence among older persons.' American Journal of Epidemiology 161, 6, 575–584. Accessed on 29/11/2019 at https://academic.oup.com/aje/article/161/6/575/80933CARE.

21   The National Academies of Sciences (2002) The Dynamics of Disability: Measuring and Monitoring Disability for Social Security Programs. Accessed on 29/11/2019 at http://nationalacademies.org/hmd/Reports/2002/The-Dynamics-of-Disability-Measuring-and-Monitoring-Disability-for-Social-Security-Programs.aspx.

22   Hardy, S.E. and Gill, T.M. (2004) 'Recovery from disability among community-dwelling older persons.' JAMA 291, 13, 1596–1602. Accessed on 29/11/2019 at www.ncbi.nlm.nih.gov/pubmed/15069047.

23   NHS (n.d.) 'Quick Guide: Discharge to Assess.' Accessed on 29/11/2019 at www.nhs.uk/NHSEngland/keogh-review/Documents/quick-guides/Quick-Guide-discharge-to-access.pdf.

24   NHS (n.d.) 'Act Now – getting people "Home First".' Accessed on 29/11/2019 at www.england.nhs.uk/wp-content/uploads/2018/12/3-grab-guide-getting-people-home-first-v2.pdf

25   The UKHCA, a provider association, offers more information about homecare: www.ukhca.co.uk.

26   Cunningham, C. (2011) 'Systemic inflammation and delirium: Important co-factors in the progression of dementia.' Biochemical Society Transactions 39, 4, 945–953. Accessed on 29/11/2019 at www.ncbi.nlm.nih.gov/pubmed/21787328.

27   Beavers, K.M., Brinkley, T.E. and Nicklas, B.J. (2010) 'Effect of exercise training on chronic inflammation.' Clinica Chimica Acta 411, 11–12, 785–793. Accessed on 29/11/2019 at www.ncbi.nlm.nih.gov/pmc/articles/PMC3629815.

28   Bellelli, G., Moresco, R., Panina-Bordignon, P., Arosio, B. et al. (2017) 'Is delirium the cognitive harbinger of frailty in older adults? A review about the existing evidence.' Frontiers in Medicine 4, 188. Accessed on 29/11/2019 at www.ncbi.nlm.nih.gov/pmc/articles/PMC5682301.

29   Page, V. and Casarin, A. (2014) 'Missing link or not, mobilise against delirium.' Critical Care 18, 105. Accessed on 29/11/2019 at https://ccforum.biomedcentral.com/articles/10.1186/cc13712.

30   Cornwell, J., Levenson, R., Sonola, L. and Poteliakhoff, E. (2012) 'Continuity of care for older hospital patients: A call for action.' The King's Fund. Accessed on 29/11/2019 at www.kingsfund.org.uk/sites/default/files/field/field_publication_file/continuity-of-care-for-older-hospital-patients-mar-2012.pdf.

31   LaHue, S.C., Douglas, V.C., Kuo, T., Conell, C.A. et al. (2019) 'Association between inpatient delirium and hospital readmission in patients ≥ 65 years of age: A retrospective cohort study.' British Journal of Hospital Medicine 14, 4, 201–206. Accessed on 29/11/2019 www.ncbi.nlm.nih.gov/pmc/articles/PMC6628723.

32   Nikelski, A., Keller, A., Schumacher-Schönert, F., Dehl, T. *et al.* (2019) 'Supporting elderly people with cognitive impairment during and after hospital stays with intersectoral care management: Study protocol for a randomized controlled trial.' *Trials 20*, 543. Accessed on 29/11/2019 https://trialsjournal.biomedcentral.com/articles/10.1186/s13063-019-3636-5.

33   Dharmarajan, K., Swami, S., Gou, R.Y., Jones, R.N. and Inouye, S.K. (2017) 'Pathway from delirium to death: Potential in-hospital mediators of excess mortality.' *Journal of the American Geriatrics Society 65*, 5, 1026–1033. Accessed on 29/11/2019 at www.ncbi.nlm.nih.gov/pubmed/28039852.

34   McCusker, J., Cole, M., Abrahamowicz, M., Primeau, F. and Belzile, E. (2002) 'Delirium predicts 12-month mortality.' *Archives of Internal Medicine 162*, 5, 457–463. Accessed on 29/11/2019 at www.ncbi.nlm.nih.gov/pubmed/11863480

35   Uno, H., Tarara, R., Else, J.G., Suleman, M.A. and Sapolsky, R.M. (1089) 'Hippocampal damage associated with prolonged and fatal stress in primates.' *Journal of Neuroscience 9*, 5, 1705–1711. Accessed on 29/11/2019 at www.jneurosci.org/content/9/5/1705.

36   Avelino-Silva, T.J., Campora, F., Curiati, J.A.E. and Jacob-Filho, W. (2018) 'Prognostic effects of delirium motor subtypes in hospitalized older adults: A prospective cohort study.' *PLOS One 13*, 1, e0191092. Accessed on 29/11/2019 at www.ncbi.nlm.nih.gov/pubmed/29381733.

37   Todd, A., Blackley, S., Burton, J.K., Stott, D.J. *et al.* (2017) 'Reduced level of arousal and increased mortality in adult acute medical admissions: A systematic review and meta-analysis.' *BMC Geriatrics 17*, 1, 283. Accessed on 29/11/2019 at www.ncbi.nlm.nih.gov/pmc/articles/PMC5721682.

9

The delirium experience

With Mark Hudson

LEARNING OBJECTIVES

When you've met one person who has survived delirium, you have only met one person who has survived delirium. But asking about the experience of someone who has been through delirium is not only interesting in terms of thinking about how the quality of care might be improved, but also is potentially informative about the underlying biological substrates. Above all, patients and carers deserve to be carefully listened to, and this chapter introduces some of the rationale for taking their stories seriously.

One patient said: 'Being a patient in Critical Care is like chucking a hand grenade into your life – it blows everything apart.'[1]

Introduction

People with lived experience are a brilliant resource for catalysing change in social movements.[2]

People with lived experience are at the heart of social movements. Their perspectives of having experienced a particular service-demand of healthcare or having faced a gap in healthcare provision often motivate a movement to begin and persist. Good person-centred care is integral to ensuring a positive experience.

There is a need for continued engagement between everyone during delirium episodes in order to use experience to influence current and future care giving. But the delirium episode is potentially very dehumanising, leading to patients and carers feeling demotivated and lacking agency, because of an increased state of dependence. Even when staff attempt to highlight the case of a delirious patient, this discourse is dominated by a biomedical and scientific narrative that serves to devalue their potential unique contribution to patient care.

The sudden and dramatic nature of their loved one's absence during delirium radically affects the lives of family members emotionally; it tends to be shocking, unexpected and distressing.

There has been a range of consistent conclusions in enquiring about the 'delirium experience'. For example, staff, patients and family experiences of giving and receiving care during an episode of delirium in an acute hospital care setting have been investigated by Health Improvement Scotland,[3] and have been invaluable in shedding light on the experiences of giving and receiving care when a person has an episode of delirium.

Some key themes can be identified as follows:

- feeling safe

- knowing the person

- being calm

- being 'kept in the loop'

- helping people make sense of things

- raising the profile of delirium.

Other specific aspects tend to emerge in probing about the 'delirium experience', including incomprehensible experiences, vivid/dramatic memories, neuropsychiatric phenomena and disorientation in time and place. Feelings of imprisonment, restraint and being trapped are also often described, and to some extent might be footed in reality.

'Experts by experience'

It is important not to underestimate patients' thinking during the delirium experience and analysis of the experience afterwards. A consultant anaesthetist recently shared in a scientific paper:[4]

It was also surprising how much I was thinking. Even if the basic assumption was paranoia, I was doing a lot of rational thinking in the situation.

Another 'survivor' describes:[5]

Totally on my own with nobody to help, it was the most traumatic episode of my life. It has left a deep emotional scar that still hurts years later.

He then says:

> Delirium is a true, actual and powerful experience and to say it is merely
> imagined, or that the patient is confused, is to severely diminish the
> significance of the condition. I was sometimes perplexed, but I 'knew' things
> were actually happening. I was not confused.

Capturing healthcare experiences is proving an effective and powerful way
of making sure that improvement of services is actually geared towards the
needs of the people using them. All experiences are valid and valuable.

'Experts by experience' are a crucial component of any work to improve
services by amplifying the voice of the people who use those services.
Understanding the difference between these experts' actual experience of
care and what they had hoped to experience defines an important 'gap' for
improvement science.

Assessments of quality of care from the patient perspective have noticeably
shifted in nuance from 'patient satisfaction' to 'patient experiences',[6] and the
term 'expert by experience' is not without controversy. Patient experience
could also be an additional, valuable source of information about safety
issues once systematically gathered and reviewed.[7]

The existent literature[8] indicates that it is not only feasible to involve
patients in the delivery or redesign of healthcare but also that such
engagement can potentially lead to a number of desirable outcomes,
including reduced hospital admissions, efficiency and quality of health
services, improved quality of life and enhanced quality of health provision.

The importance of stories

Listen to a story of anyone who has experienced delirium whenever you can.

Narratives, also referred to as 'storytelling' and testimonials, are particularly
compelling because they are easily understandable and memorable. Narratives
can facilitate 'making sense' of the environment and provide value and
emotional appeal to the information provided. People often relate to narrative
information regardless of their level of literacy or culture.

Messages can 'connect' with people, because they resonate with a
particular emotional picture. These messages then have the potential to
engage people and change behaviour. As articulated by Don Berwick when
he was leading the Institute for Healthcare Improvement, 'the value of
storytelling in healthcare is immense and virtually untapped'.[9]

Exploring stories of survivors of delirium might even help to identify
the underlying neural substrates. Although it is conceded that delirium

is not simply a collection of 'dreams', the science of dreaming potentially constitutes a relevant topic in contemporary neuroscience and provides major insights into the study of human consciousness.[10] There might be similarities between the experiences of delirium and 'lucid dreaming' in terms of the neural networks engaged. Whether experiences best resemble 'dreams' or psychosis is a fascinating area, which relies on good reports of experiences.[11]

Table 9.1 describes some models relevant to narratives.

Table 9.1 Description of some models relevant to narratives

Model	Description
Elaboration likelihood model[12]	This model is about persuasion and attitude change. In this model, it's proposed that there are two 'routes': central and peripheral. In the central route, the person makes his mind up on a careful analysis of the merits of the case. In the peripheral route, the person is able to make his mind up on the basis of positive and negative cues related to the stimulus.
Transportation models[13]	A person is able to engage with a story if he is able to empathise with some of the characters or context. Transportation models explain how listeners 'lose' themselves in a story.
Entertainment overcoming resistance model[14]	In this model, when listeners are engaged within the story or when they relate to characters similar to themselves, they change their attitude and behaviour because they are less likely to resist the story.
Kahneman's two-system way of thinking[15]	Kahneman distinguishes essentially between two systems of thinking: 'System 1' (Thinking Fast) is the intuitive way of thinking and making decisions, fast and instinctive, whereas 'System 2' (Thinking Slow) is the analytical way of making decisions, slow and deliberative.

There is currently an emphasis on the provision of patient-centred care in all aspects of healthcare in order to improve the patent and carer experience. In order to enter into a therapeutic relationship with a patient, clinicians must first develop an understanding of their own beliefs, concerns, values and expectations, and their ability to create relationships before they can respond to the needs of patients.

Therapeutic relationships can deteriorate in any place and at any time. Examples of this include:

- between carers and staff
- between carers and the patient
- between carers themselves.

In a qualitative study of 'terminal restlessness',[16] disagreements and tension between staff and carers were reported, which arose fundamentally from differing understandings of the patient's needs. The carer–patient relationship also suffers as carers experience the loss of a loved and familiar person before their actual physical death.

Carers

Delirium is very distressing to carers, both unpaid and paid, potentially increasing the risk of adverse psychological outcomes. The family is an important target in care, and, in delirium, clinicians should provide care to family members, not only patients who may lack mental capacity while experiencing delirium. Care strategies can include: reassuring the families that they could safely leave the patients' care to the staff, making the hospital environment comfortable for the families especially 'after hours', and coordinating support from involved parties. It is important that friends and family have an opportunity for 'debriefing' about the delirium episode.

As has been emphasised throughout this book, delirium is described as a psychologically traumatic experience, not only for patients, but also for their families and nurses caring for them.

Qualitative research shows that the experience of delirium as changes or failure to recognise loved ones is profoundly frightening for carers. Education about delirium may help family members to recognise the symptoms of delirium so that they are less uncertain and fearful when episodes occur, and to help to adopt appropriate attitudes regarding delirium.[17]

The 'burden' from delirium needs to be acknowledged; it includes significant and sustained emotional and psychological impact of witnessing delirium. Burden might legitimately considered an important outcome for clinical trials and other intervention studies for delirium. Delirium burden on family carers can be evaluated using the DEL-B-C instrument.[18]

Distress in delirium

There are many reasons for a person to become distressed (see Figure 9.1). The causes are not only psychological causes but include identifiable physical causes.

Causes of distress in people with delirium

Pain	Loneliness	Fear
Delusions	Thirst, hunger	Constipation
Hallucinations	Urinary retention	Unpredictable, unfamiliar environment
Loss of control	Feeling confined	Noise

Figure 9.1 Causes of distress

Reproduced by kind permission of Prof. Alasdair MacLullich.

Resilience is an ill-defined concept, and its relation to delirium is currently not understood well. Family member distress occurs no matter how healthy or 'resilient' families are, because reciprocal long-lasting relationships and a clear individuated personality appear to be lost temporarily. NICE clinical guidelines advocate the involvement of carers in the management of patients with delirium and recommend that information and support in relation to delirium should be offered to them.[19]

Although distress after recovery from delirium is an important consequence of delirium, it has perhaps not received as much attention as it should have. The question of the extent to which there are commonalities in distress across different care settings and across different primary diagnoses remains unresolved as yet.

Negative emotions

Specific **negative emotions** include fear, embarrassment, anger, hopelessness, insecurity and guilt. Some carers experience the patient's behaviour as 'unnatural' and 'frightening', particularly if the patient became aggressive during the delirium episode.[20] There is a consistently reported blurring of reality.

Guilt often occurs when carers feel they have not been able to better care for the patient. Not knowing the cause of delirium is also frightening for carers. Others might be 'embarrassed' by the patient's actions during delirium, especially in the presence of others. Anger, frustration and disappointment can be experienced by carers when they could no longer have a meaningful interaction with the patient, and carers feel sadness relating to the changes in the patient in the sense of 'anticipatory grief'.

Memory for the delirium episode

It has been reported that a majority of patients can recall their delirium experience, and that a majority of patients view their delirium experience as 'distressing'.[21] Delirium is a condition that can be frightening for those directly experiencing it, as well as anyone witnessing it.

In one study,[22] it was reported that the majority of those who could not remember being 'confused' were not distressed, and most of those patients who remembered that they were confused had a mild level of distress. Differences in distress severity could conceivably be due to clinical and psychological factors, such as severity of an underlying physical illness and the pre-morbid personality traits of the patient.

Several published papers have reported that moderate to severe levels of distress are experienced by the majority of carers of patients with delirium, but there are a number of variables, such as the type of delirium, identity of underlying diagnosis, and support networks of carers.[23] Patient markers of carer distress include poor physical performance status, the presence of hyperactive delirium, hallucinations, agitation, cognitive decline and incoherent speech.[24]

Among the various symptoms of delirium, in those who can recall their experience and who report distress about their experience, recalled phenomena have included 'those of insomnia, followed by visual hallucinations, uncooperativeness for treatment, pulling out tubes, and being abusive'.[25] Perceptual disturbances, including visual, auditory and olfactory hallucinations, have been reported, including seeing small animals, insects and strangers.

Critical care experience

Patients with ICU delirium have been historically excluded from research for reasons such as perceived lack of communication or lack of cooperation. The critical care setting may expose family members to a variety of stressors, such as communication problems, uncertainty about future prognosis and lack of support for shared decisions.

Some possible reactions of patients with ICU delirium might include:[26]

- a feeling of fear – e.g. in relation to falling asleep, perceived jeopardy of personal safety, and/or perceived helplessness

- a feeling of being disconnected or feeling of being separated from others, and the need to relate emotionally and physically in the ICU environment

- difficulty in differentiating between what was real or not.

A personal account of ICU delirium

Optimising long-term outcomes for survivors of critical illness must begin with a discussion of the patient's experience in the setting of critical illness. This, from Mark Hudson, is a real account, and to include it here is an honour.

My name is Mark Hudson and I am an ICU delirium survivor. I was admitted to my local hospital's ICU on 27 December 2015 and when I returned to the world it was the middle of January 2016. In this time, I experienced ICU delirium, and I did not wish to pass up this opportunity to help raise understanding of this little spoken about medical condition.

So, to give a little context to what will follow, I will share with you a few parts of my delirium and what I think helped to precipitate them. Like a lot of delirium sufferers, I felt in constant danger, I was being hunted down and tortured – one of the main ways they tortured me was to slit open my wrists and let me bleed. Barbaric, I know, but where I was cut in my delirium coincided with where the arterial lines were placed; as my brain was unable to understand what was going on, it interpreted what was going on itself. I was dying and something was happening to me, happening without my knowledge and without my consent; I was being tortured. That was the only logical conclusion.

The second was the fact I had acute respiratory distress syndrome (ARDS) which causes the lungs to become inflamed and liquid to leak into the lungs. While ventilated, things are OK as the oxygen is getting into your blood even if it is forced into it. However, you can't be ventilated for ever, so to help you wean off the vent they do what they call sprints. Sprints, as I understand it, involve reducing how much work the ventilator is doing for your lungs, making you work a bit to breathe so your breathing muscles can re-strengthen. But what a patient with delirium experiences is a sudden ability not to be able to breathe properly and an awareness of fluid in their lungs. How does the brain understand these things without context? You are drowning. This was the other main form of torture in my delirious state.

These are simplified parts of my delirium, I was in a constant state of fear, a fear brought on by perhaps a biological understanding that I was near death. A fear made worse by the very things the excellent doctors did to save my life. As one of my ICU consultants told me, in any other setting what we do would be torture but because we do it to save your life it is OK. And this is very true, and it is certainly not something we can change in an ICU setting. But how can we reduce its effects? The answer is to me very simple: understanding – understanding that what you do, even if the patient is unaware, will affect them. It might affect them in ways you don't understand or realise until much later. The only way to tackle delirium effectively is to understand the effect it has on a person, to grasp that the person retreating into themselves post-op might actually be in a living nightmare. That patient screaming and shouting might be doing so because they think you're trying to poison them. When context and understanding is placed over a person's actions, then what seems to be strange actions becomes clear.

A patient's experience is vital in all aspects of medicine as they are the people who will be the recipients of the treatments. We are also the people who have experienced the current treatments and understand the conditions in a way most doctors will never have to. So, to move forward with better treatments, strategies and protocols, we need to work together, healthcare professionals and patients, making things better for everyone who comes after us.

Endnotes

1   NHS University Hospitals Plymouth (2019) 'Intensive care rehabilitation team named regional champion in prestigious award.' Accessed on 29/11/2019 at www.plymouthhospitals.nhs.uk/latest-news/intensive-care-rehabilitation-team-shortlisted-for-prestigious-award--3023.

2   del Castillo, J., Nicholas, L., Nye, R. and Khan, H. (2017) 'We change the world: What can we learn from global social movements for health?' *Nesta.* Accessed on 29/11/2019 at https://media.nesta.org.uk/documents/we_change_the_world_report.pdf, p.6.

3   Health Improvement Scotland (2013) 'Think Delirium: Staff, patients and families experiences of giving and receiving care during an episode of delirium in an acute hospital care setting.' Accessed on 29/11/2019 at www.kingsfund.org.uk/sites/default/files/media/Healthcare%20Improvement%20 Scotland,%20Improving%20Older%20People's%20Acute%20Care%20in%20NHS%20Scotland%20 -%20staff%20report.pdf

4   Larsen, R.A. (2019) 'Just a little delirium – A report from the other side.' *Anaesthesiologica Scandinavica* 63, 8, 1095–1096. Accessed on 29/11/2019 at https://onlinelibrary.wiley.com/doi/full/10.1111/aas.13416.

5   Garrett, R.M. (2019) 'Reflections on delirium – A patient's perspective.' *Journal of the Intensive Care Society.* Accessed on 29/11/2019 at https://journals.sagepub.com/doi/full/10.1177/1751143719851352.

6   NHS Confederation (2010) *Feeling Better? Improving Patient Experience in Hospital.* Accessed on 29/11/2019 at www.nhsconfed.org/~/media/Confederation/Files/Publications/Documents/Feeling_better_Improving_patient_experience_in_hospital_Report.pdf

7   NIHR Signal (2019) 'Communication problems are top of patients' concerns about hospital care.' Accessed on 29/11/2019 at https://discover.dc.nihr.ac.uk/content/signal-000758/communication-problems-are-top-of-patients-concerns-about-hospital-care.

8   Bombard, Y., Baker, G.R., Orlando, E., Fancott, C. *et al.* (2018) 'Engaging patients to improve quality of care: A systematic review.' *Implementation Science 31,* 1, 98. Accessed on 29/11/2019 at www.ncbi.nlm.nih.gov/pubmed/30045735.

9   Grissinger, M. (2014) 'Telling true stories is an ISMP hallmark: Here's why you should tell stories, too...' *Pharmacy and Therapeutics 39,* 10, 658–659. Accessed on 29/11/2019 at www.ncbi.nlm.nih.gov/pmc/articles/PMC4189689.

10   Mutz, J. and Amir-Homayoun, J. (2017) 'Exploring the neural correlates of dream phenomenonology and altered states of consciousness during sleep.' *Neuroscience of Consciousness 2017,* 1, nix009. Accessed on 29/11/2019 at www.ncbi.nlm.nih.gov/pmc/articles/PMC6007136.

11   See e.g. the account by Matthew d'Ancona: https://members.tortoisemedia.com/2019/08/13/delirium-tremendous/content.html?sig=yqBcIiR32APsEV5WcIVZi5EJk5wQchd2-FkgZU9zs6A.

12   See e.g. Petty, R.E. and Cacioppo, J.T. (1986) 'The Elaboration Likelihood Model of persuasion.' *Advances in Experimental Social Psychology 19,* 123–205, Accessed on 16/12/2019 at www.sciencedirect.com/science/article/pii/S0065260108602142.

13   See e.g. Isberner, M.-B., Richter, T., Schreiner, C., Eisenbach, Y., Sommer, C., and Appel, M. (2018) 'Empowering stories: Transportation into narratives with strong protagonists increases self-related control beliefs.' *Discourse Processes 56,* 8, 575–598. Accessed on 16/12/2019 at www.tandfonline.com/doi/full/10.1080/0163853X.2018.1526032.

14   See e.g. Fransen, M.L., Smit, E.G. and Verlegh, P.W.J. (2015) 'Strategies and motives for resistance to persuasion: An integrative framework.' *Frontiers in Psychology 6,* 1201. Accessed on 16/12/2019 at www.ncbi.nlm.nih.gov/pmc/articles/PMC4536373.

15   See e.g. Kahneman, D. (2012) 'Of 2 minds: How fast and slow thinking shape perception and choice (excerpt).' *Scientific American.* Accessed on 16/12/2019 at www.scientificamerican.com/article/kahneman-excerpt-thinking-fast-and-slow.

16   Brajtman, S. (2005) 'Terminal restlessness: Perspectives of an interdisciplinary palliative care team.' *International Journal of Palliative Nursing 11*, 4, 172–178. Accessed on 29/11/2019 at www.ncbi.nlm. nih.gov/pubmed/15924033.

17   Carbone, M.K. and Gugliucci, M.R. (2015) 'Delirium and the family caregiver: The need for evidence-based education interventions.' *Gerontologist 55*, 3, 345–352. Accessed on 29/11/2019 at www.ncbi.nlm. nih.gov/pubmed/24847844.

18   Racine, A.M., D'Aquila, M., Schmitt, E.M, Gallagher, J. *et al.* (2018) 'Delirium burden in patients and family caregivers: Development and testing of new instruments.' *Gerontologist*, doi: 10.1093/geront/gny041. Accessed on 29/11/2019 at www.ncbi.nlm.nih.gov/pubmed/29746694.

19   National Institute for Health and Care Excellence (2018) 'Dementia: Assessment, management and support for people living with dementia and their carers.' NICE guideline [NG97]. www.nice.org.uk/guidance/ng97/chapter/Recommendations.

20   Finucane, A.M., Lugton, J., Kennedy, C. and Spiller, J.A. (2017) 'The experiences of caregivers of patients with delirium, and their role in its management in palliative care settings: An integrative literature review.' *Psycho-Oncology 26*, 3, 291–300. Accessed on 29/11/2019 at www.ncbi.nlm.nih.gov/pmc/articles/PMC5363350.

21   Breitbart, W., Gibson, C. and Tremblay, A. (2002) 'The delirium experience: Delirium recall and delirium-related distress in hospitalized patients with cancer, the spouses/caregivers, and their nurses.' *Psychosomatics 43*, 3, 183–194. Accessed on 28/11/2019 at www.ncbi.nlm.nih.gov/pubmed/12075033.

22   Grover, S., Ghosh, A. and Ghormode, D. (2015) 'Experience in delirium: Is it distressing?' *Journal of Neuropsychiatry and Clinical Neurosciences 27*, 139–146. Accessed on 28/11/2019 at https://neuro.psychiatryonline.org/doi/pdfplus/10.1176/appi.neuropsych.13110329.

23   Finucane, A.M., Lugton, J., Kennedy, C. and Spiller, J.A. (2017) 'The experiences of caregivers of patients with delirium, and their role in its management in palliative care settings: Ain integrative literature review.' *Psycho-Oncology 26*, 3, 291–300. Accessed on 28/11/2019 at www.ncbi.nlm.nih.gov/pmc/articles/PMC5363350/#pon4140-bib-0025.

24   Finucane, A.M., Lugton, J., Kennedy, C. and Spiller, J.A. (2017) 'The experiences of caregivers of patients with delirium, and their role in its management in palliative care settings: Ain integrative literature review.' *Psycho-Oncology 26*, 3, 291–300. Accessed on 28/11/2019 at www.ncbi.nlm.nih.gov/pmc/articles/PMC5363350/#pon4140-bib-0025.

25   Grover, S., Ghosh, A. and Ghormode, D. (2015) 'Experience in delirium: Is it distressing?' *Journal of Neuropsychiatry and Clinical Neurosciences 27*, 139–146. Accessed on 28/11/2019 at https://neuro.psychiatryonline.org/doi/pdfplus/10.1176/appi.neuropsych.13110329.

26   Gaete Ortega, D., Papathanassoglou, E. and Norris, C.M. (2019) 'The lived experience of delirium in intensive care unit patients: A meta-ethnography.' *Australian Critical Care*. doi: 10.1016/j.aucc.2019.01.003. Accessed on 28/11/2019 at www.ncbi.nlm.nih.gov/pubmed/30871853.

10

Law, ethics and safeguarding in delirium care

LEARNING OBJECTIVES

Delirium care ultimately takes place within the constraints of legal and ethical frameworks which vary across jurisdictions. This chapter will introduce you to some of the issues raised by the lack of mental capacity, but also encourage you to think about how human rights approaches are reconciled with the care actually provided.

This chapter concentrates on the law currently operating in England and Wales.

Whenever competing rights are involved, or if someone is in danger, the law gets involved. Good health and social care for the vulnerable is a moral, ethical and legal imperative. Adults considered to be unable to make a particular decision or take a particular action for themselves at the time the decision or action needs to be taken, due to an impairment or disturbance in the functioning of the mind or brain, are described as **lacking decision-making capacity**.

How duty of care contributes to safe practice

If you assume it, you have a **duty of care** to all those receiving care and support in your workplace. This means promoting wellbeing and making sure that people are kept safe from harm, abuse and injury. Wellbeing could be defined as 'a positive outcome that is meaningful for people and for many sectors of society, because it tells us that people perceive that their lives are going well.'[1]

Issues about consent relate to effective communication (the importance of which was discussed in Chapter 5) and the legal requirements for demonstrating mental capacity which is time- and decision-specific. In clinical care, consent normally involves obtaining oral informed consent before procedures, explaining the procedures before initiating them, so that patients fully understand what is proposed in their care.

Delirium, however, is complicated. Some people may have capacity to consent to some interventions but not to others, or may have capacity at some times but not others. Assessment of the patient's capacity to make decisions about health and personal care is fundamental, and must also be taken into consideration. If the person is deemed to lack mental capacity, appropriate steps must be taken.

The **GMC guidance 'Consent: patients and doctors making decisions together'** is readily available.[2] Clauses 75 and 76 are relevant to 'Making decisions when a patient lacks capacity'.

Introduction to key legislation

Up to half of patients in acute medical and psychiatric healthcare settings lack decision-making capacity, rising to around 70% in settings such as care homes and approaching 90% in intensive care settings.[3]

Delirium is a mental disorder within the meaning of the **Mental Health Act 1983** (MHA); as such, use of the Act may need to be considered if the patient decides they wish to leave the hospital. There are some potential attractions in the use of the MHA: where someone has a mental illness needing treatment alongside a physical health condition; and where the person is presenting particular risk of harm to others.

The **Mental Capacity Act 2005** (MCA) sets out a clear framework for those people who lack capacity and all significant decisions made must be in the best interests of the person. A structured capacity assessment must be undertaken at the first possible opportunity and a best interests decision properly documented. A capacity assessment should include the decision to keep a patient in hospital for investigation and treatment, and proposed interventions must be specified. Where a patient who lacks capacity needs to remain in hospital against their will for longer than 72 hours, they will need to be detained via the Deprivation of Liberty Safeguards (2007).

The MCA is based on **five key principles:**[4]

- Principle 1: A presumption of capacity.

- Principle 2: Individuals being supported to make their own decisions.

- Principle 3: Unwise decisions.

- Principle 4: Best interests.

- Principle 5: Less restrictive option.

Under the MCA, a person must be assumed to have capacity unless it is established that they lack capacity. If there is any doubt, then the healthcare professional should assess the capacity of the patient to take the decision in question. This assessment and the conclusions drawn from it should be recorded in the patient's notes. Capacity is decision- and time-specific, and may fluctuate throughout the course of an admission. Capacity arguably should be reassessed for each new decision, and the least restrictive course of action taken for the patient.

The MCA also requires that all practical and appropriate steps are taken to enable a person to make the decision themselves. These steps might include:[5]

- providing relevant information

- communicating in an appropriate way

- making the person feel at ease

- supporting the person.

The law in cases of 'fluctuating capacity' is not yet settled (see *Royal Borough of Greenwich v CDM* [2018]), as there is no legal framework for it.[6] Overly paternalistic ethical approval processes might have a detrimental effect on our ability to open up this space.

How 'best interests' decisions may need to be made for those lacking capacity

Some patients experiencing delirium may not be able to consent at that particular moment in time.

Where it has been decided that a person with dementia is unable to make a decision for themselves, care staff must do what is in the person's best interests. This is known as a 'best interests decision'.

When deciding what is in the person's best interests you need to:[7]

- involve the person in the decision as much as possible

- respect their culture, including their religious beliefs

- talk to people who know them well

- try to limit restrictions on the person.

How advance decisions can be used to provide information about the wishes of an individual

An **advance decision** (sometimes known as an advance decision to refuse treatment, an ADRT or a living will) is a decision you can make now, if you have capacity, to refuse a specific type of treatment at some time in the future. An advance decision is only legally binding as long as it complies with the MCA Code of Practice and meets a number of specific conditions. It lets your family, carers and health professionals know whether you want to refuse *specific* treatments in the future.

This means they will know your wishes if you are unable to make or communicate those decisions yourself. As long as it is valid and applies to your situation, an advance decision gives your health and social care team clinical and legal instructions about your treatment choices.

An advance decision will only be used if, at some time in the future, you are not able to make your own decisions about your treatment. It is the responsibility of the person making the advance decision to make sure the healthcare professionals treating them are aware of any decision that has been made.[8]

The importance of sharing safeguarding information with the relevant agencies

Adults have a general right to independence, choice and self-determination, including control over information about themselves. In the context of adult safeguarding, these rights can be overridden in certain circumstances. Emergency or life-threatening situations may warrant the sharing of relevant information with the relevant emergency services without consent. The law does not prevent the sharing of sensitive, personal information between organisations where the public interest served outweighs the public interest served by protecting confidentiality – for example, where a serious crime may be prevented. Patients with delirium can be at high risk of abuse across a number of domains – for instance, physical, emotional, financial – and we all need to be vigilant about their wider protection.

The **Data Protection Act 1998** enables the lawful sharing of information. There should be a local agreement or protocol in place setting out the processes and principles for sharing information between organisations.

Frontline staff and volunteers should always report safeguarding concerns in line with their organisation's policy. It is good practice to try to gain the person's consent to share information.

Deprivation of Liberty Safeguards

Deprivation of Liberty Safeguards (DoLS) were initially designed for long-term use – for example, with residents of care homes. The DoLS are part of the MCA,[9] and aim to make sure that people are looked after in a way that does not inappropriately restrict their freedom.[10]

The safeguards set out a process that hospitals and care homes must follow if they believe it is in the person's best interests to deprive that person of their liberty, by application to a local authority.[11]

Examples of making decisions or placing restriction on someone with cognitive impairment could include deciding on the person's routine, stopping them from walking about at night or preventing them from leaving. Care-home or hospital staff should make sure that all care a person receives involves as little restriction as possible. However, sometimes it will be necessary to take away some of the person's freedom to provide them with the care they need. Sometimes, taking away a person's freedom in this way can amount to a 'deprivation of liberty'.

A deprivation of liberty occurs when:[12]

> The person is under continuous supervision and control and is not free to leave, and the person lacks capacity to consent to these arrangements.

There is no statutory definition of a deprivation of liberty beyond that in the *Cheshire West* and *Surrey* Supreme Court judgement, March 2014 – the 'acid test'.[13] DoLS are strict processes that must be followed. They are a set of checks that are designed to ensure that a person who is deprived of their liberty is protected, and that this course of action is both appropriate and in the person's best interests. The definition of what counts as a deprivation of liberty is wide. DoLS nonetheless attempt to offer protection to ensure that when someone's freedom is restricted, it is both in their best interests and, where possible, done in the least restrictive way.

The key elements of these safeguards are:[14]

- to provide the person with a representative

- to give the person (or their representative) the right to challenge a deprivation of liberty through the Court of Protection

- to provide a mechanism for any deprivation of liberty to be reviewed and monitored regularly.

Deprivation of liberty (DoL) may occur if the criteria are met – that is, it is a mental disorder under the MHA,[15] a patient lacks capacity to consent, and it is in the best interests of the patient to be deprived of liberty. In practice, the delirium is likely to be sufficiently short-lived such that only an urgent authorisation will be used. Arguably, DoLS are not really set up to deal with short-term DoL or fluctuating capacity, as you can't use a second urgent authorisation later in the same period of care in the same place if the person loses capacity again.

Liberty Protection Safeguards

In 2017, the English Law Commission put forward proposals to replace DoLS with 'Liberty Protection Safeguards' (LPS).[16] This will shape Parliament's ultimate response. The Liberty Protection Safeguards are said to broaden the scope to treat people and to deprive patients of their liberty.[17] The definition of 'mental disorder' in the LPS is the same definition as under Section 1(2) of Mental Health Act 2007 and currently used under DoLS, which is 'any disorder or disability of the mind'.[18]

There are three authorisation conditions that must be met as part of the legal criteria for an authorisation:[19]

1. The 'cared-for person' lacks mental capacity.

2. They have a mental disorder.

3. The arrangements (restrictions) are necessary and proportionate.

The target date for implementation is spring 2020. Prior to then, a revised MCA Code of Practice will be published, which, the sector trusts, will bring clarity to some outstanding questions about how LPS will work in practice.

Legal powers

It is worth noting that legislations devolved to the regions of the UK exist in relation to this topic.

Legal powers are needed before making best interest decisions about the money or property of a person with cognitive impairment. It is critical to identify the family and/or main carer of the patient. Ensure that the patient's contact details are on file. If the patient lacks capacity, ascertain whether a family member or carer has Power of Attorney/Guardianship over welfare.

There are three possibilities.

Lasting Power of Attorney

Adults can give someone else the power to make decisions about their money and property. This is called making a Lasting Power of Attorney (property and affairs).

Deputy

If someone has lost capacity to make some financial decisions, an application can be made to the Court of Protection to appoint someone to look after their money.

Appointee

The Department for Work and Pensions can appoint someone else to receive a patient's benefits and to use that money to pay for expenses such as household bills, food, personal items and residential accommodation charges. Appointees can only make decisions about the money received in benefits.

Vulnerability

Vulnerability is a complex concept in the law; for example, the **Safeguarding Vulnerable Groups Act 2006**[20] broadly defines vulnerability in terms of receiving care or treatment, or specific place of residence, but also considers age, health status and disability.

In the broadest sense, adults can be defined as vulnerable because they are receiving health and/or social care, but more specifically delirium can make a person increasingly vulnerable. Cognitive impairment increases vulnerability as it compromises effective rational decision-making.

Informed consent and mental capacity

Informed consent is an issue within medical ethics that is constantly in evolution and under analysis on both philosophical and jurisprudence grounds. Historically, the effects of certain medical conditions have often been conveniently used as a pretext for paternalism in medical practice; the beneficence and non-maleficence models of medical ethics have long dominated the approach to treatment. But in delirium this paternalism, especially in a mistaken belief that a patient may be imminently dying, might lead to excessive end-of-life investigations.[21]

Reasons for adopting a human rights approach

A human rights-based approach to care establishes minimum standards of care, a legal and regulatory threshold, that help to safeguard individuals, particularly those who are vulnerable. It may overlap with a person-centred approach.

Rights-based approaches promote human rights and personhood. It is acknowledged that caring for a patient with delirium can also impact negatively on staff's emotions. Most of the work examining this explores the impact of delirium on nursing staff as they tend to be most frequently and closely in contact with patients.

Arguably, we need a human rights-based approach because such an approach:

- respects diversity, promoting equality and ensuring human rights

- speaks to the values of practitioners and professionals in delirium care.

The World Health Organization highlights that people with cognitive impairment are vulnerable to having their human rights overlooked and therefore need to have their dignity respected in all settings and contexts. Several healthcare 'scandals' in England have especially highlighted the importance of creating the right culture of care to ensure that people are treated in ways that promote dignity and respect. Public sector bodies have duties to respect, protect and fulfil the rights that people have under the **Human Rights Act 1998**, and this includes regulators of health and social care. There are also duties to eliminate discrimination and advance equality of opportunity, and to foster good relations between different groups, under the **Equality Act 2010**.

People with cognitive impairments, including those with dementia and delirium, have traditionally been among the most devalued in our society. This has led to care practices that undermine the humanity and personhood of individuals with dementia.

Physical restraints

The use of physical restraint is controversial. In legal and ethical terms, the use of bedrails, or even covert restraint such as the tactical positioning of furniture, infringes the autonomy and dignity of patients—and is therefore maleficent.

Restraint may be defined as 'the intentional restriction of a person's voluntary movement or behaviour',[22] and may be context-dependent. Bedrails used to stop a patient purposefully leaving their bed may constitute restraint, but if used to prevent an accidental fall from bed, may not be restraint. Restraint has been defined in the legislation, but is subject to conditions to justify its use. The distinction between the interpretation of the terms 'restriction' and 'deprivation' is complex.[23]

The MCA does not state what duration and frequency of restraint would constitute a deprivation of liberty.[24]

Some beds may not comply with dimensional standards to minimise entrapment risks. This emphasises the need for careful selection of patients for whom bedrails are to be used as well as the need for monitoring and maintenance of bed systems.[25] Arguments against using bedrails include that they are ineffective in preventing falls and that they are inherently dangerous.

Involuntary antipsychotic medications

Involuntary treatment with antipsychotic medication poses a very difficult legal and ethical problem because of the widely accepted notion that the patient, not the physician or other care provider, is empowered to make decisions about whether a medical treatment will be administered.

Excited delirium and the 'excessive use of force'

Excited delirium syndrome (ExDS) was first introduced in Chapter 1. Over the past few years, the association between police coercion methods and cases of in-custody deaths have attracted the attention of the media and contributed to public opinion about ExDS. Many of incidents involve a person with ExDS who is behaving in a bizarre fashion, is restrained by the police and subsequently dies during or immediately after a struggle. Causes of death have often been attributed to positional asphyxiation, traumatic asphyxiation and less-than-lethal weapons.[26] How the law treats patients with ExDS fairly is a matter of grave concern.

Endnotes

1   Centers for Disease Control and Prevention (2018) 'Well-Being Concepts.' Accessed on 28/11/2019 at www.cdc.gov/hrqol/wellbeing.htm.

2   General Medical Council (2008) 'Consent: Patients and doctors making decisions together.' Accessed on 28/11/2019 at www.gmc-uk.org/-/media/documents/consent---english-0617_pdf-48903482.pdf.

3   Shepherd, V., Wood, F., Griffith, R., Sheehan, M. and Hood, K. (2019) 'Protection by exclusion? The (lack of) inclusion in adults who lack capacity to consent to research in clinical trials in the UK.' Trials 20, 474. Accessed on 28/11/2019 at https://trialsjournal.biomedcentral.com/articles/10.1186/s13063-019-3603 1.

4   Social Care Institute for Excellence (2016) 'Mental Capacity Act 2005 at a glance.' Accessed on 29/11/2019 at www.scie.org.uk/mca/introduction/mental-capacity-act-2005-at-a-glance.

5   Based on Department of Health and Social Care (2009) 'Reference guide to consent for examination or treatment (second edition).' Accessed on 29/11/2019 at www.gov.uk/government/publications/reference-guide-to-consent-for-examination-or-treatment-second-edition.

6   England and Wales Court of Protection Decisions: Royal Borough of Greenwich v CDM [2018] EWCOP 15 (29 June 2018). Accessed on 29/11/2019 at www.bailii.org/ew/cases/EWCOP/2018/15.html.

7   Social Care Institute for Excellence (2015) 'Making decisions in a person's best interests.' Accessed on 29/11/2019 at www.scie.org.uk/dementia/supporting-people-with-dementia/decisions/best-interest.asp.

8   Medical Protection (2015) 'Mental Capacity Act 2005 – Advance decisions.' Accessed on 29/11/2019 at www.medicalprotection.org/uk/articles/advance-decisions.

9   Mental Capacity Act 2005. Accessed on 29/11/2019 at www.legislation.gov.uk/ukpga/2005/9/contents.

10   Social Care Institute for Excellence (2017) 'Deprivation of Liberty Safeguards (DoLS) at a glance.' Accessed on 29/11/2019 at www.scie.org.uk/mca/dols/at-a-glance.

11   Parker, R., Thake, M., Attar, S., Barker, J. and Hubbard, I. (2015) 'Deprivation of liberty: A practical guide.' *GM: Supporting Healthcare Professionals in 50+ Medicine 2*. Accessed on 29/11/2019 at www.gmjournal.co.uk/deprivation-of-liberty-apractical-guide.

12   Age UK (2019) 'Factsheet 62: Deprivation of Liberty Safeguards.' Accessed on 29/11/2019 at www.ageuk.org.uk/globalassets/age-uk/documents/factsheets/fs62_deprivation_of_liberty_safeguards_fcs.pdf.

13   Judgement: *P (by his litigation friend the Official Solicitor) (Appellant) v Cheshire West and Chester Council and another (Respondents); P and Q (by their litigation friend the Official Solicitor) (Appellants) v Surrey County Council (Respondent)*. Accessed on 29/11/2019 at www.supremecourt.uk/cases/docs/uksc-2012-0068-judgment.pdf.

14   Alzheimer's Society (n.d.) 'Deprivation of Liberty Safeguards (DoLS).' Accessed on 29/11/2019 at www.alzheimers.org.uk/get-support/legal-financial/deprivation-liberty-safeguards-dols.

15   Mental Health Act 1983. Accessed on 29/11/2019 at www.legislation.gov.uk/ukpga/1983/20/contents.

16   House of Commons and House of Lords Joint Committee on Human Rights (2018) 'The Right to Freedom and Safety: Reform of the Deprivation of Liberty Safeguards.' Accessed on 29/11/2019 at https://publications.parliament.uk/pa/jt201719/jtselect/jtrights/890/890.pdf.

17   Social Care Institute for Excellence (2019) 'Liberty Protection Safeguards (LPS).' Accessed on 29/11/2019 at www.scie.org.uk/mca/dols/practice/lps.

18   Mental Health Act 2007, Chapter 12. Accessed on 29/11/2019 at www.legislation.gov.uk/ukpga/2007/12/pdfs/ukpga_20070012_en.pdf.

19   Edge Training (2019) 'Liberty Protection Safeguards (LPS): Jargon Buster.' Accessed on 29/11/2019 at www.edgetraining.org.uk/wp-content/uploads/2019/06/LPS_Jargon_Buster_June_2019.pdf.

20   Thomson Reuters Practical Law (2019) 'Safeguarding Vulnerable Groups Act 2006.' Accessed on 1/12/2019 at https://uk.practicallaw.thomsonreuters.com/7-500-6748?transitionType=Default&contextData=(sc.Default)&firstPage=true&bhcp=1.

21   Cardona-Morell, M., Kim, J.C.H., Turner, R.M., Anstey, M., Mitchell, I.A. and Hillman, K. (2016) 'Non-beneficial treatments in hospital at the end of life: A systematic review on extent of the problem.' *International Journal for Quality in Health Care 28*, 4, 456–469. Accessed on 1/12/2019 at https://academic.oup.com/intqhc/article/28/4/456/2594949.

22   College of Paramedics (2013) 'The National Ambulance Mental health group.' Accessed on 1/12/2019 at www.collegeofparamedics.co.uk/news/the-national-ambulance-mental-health-group.

23   Gupta, N. (2009) 'Complexities related to Deprivation of Liberty Safeguards and Mental Capacity Act in general hospital settings.' *BMJ 338*, b1888. Accessed on 2/12/2019 at www.bmj.com/rapid-response/2011/11/02/complexities-related-deprivation-liberty-safeguards-and-mental-capacity-ac.

24   Parker, R., Thake, M., Attar, S., Barker, J. and Hubbard, I. (2015) 'Deprivation of liberty: A practical guide.' *GM: Supporting Healthcare Professionals in 50+ Medicine 2*. Accessed on 2/12/2019 at www.gmjournal.co.uk/deprivation-of-liberty-apractical-guide.

25   Haugh, J., O Flatharta, T., Griffin, T.P. and O'Keeffe, S.T. (2014) 'High frequency of potential entrapment gaps in beds in an acute hospital.' *Age and Ageing 43*, 6, 862–865. Accessed on 2/12/2019 at www.ncbi.nlm.nih.gov/pubmed/25012157.

26   Kennedy, D.B. and Savard, D.M. (2017) 'Delayed in-custody death involving excited delirium.' *Journal of Correctional Health Care 24*, 1, 43–51. Accessed on 2/12/2019 at https://journals.sagepub.com/doi/full/10.1177/1078345817726085

11

Palliative and end-of-life care, and delirium

LEARNING OBJECTIVES

Delirium is very common in palliative care. As this is such a huge field, this chapter will only introduce you to some of the topics that are important in palliative care to do with delirium. These include the detection of delirium, palliative sedation, processes and approaches during 'end-of-life' or dying, reversibility, conversations around dying, whether the construct of a 'good death' applies to delirium, and promoting high-quality research.

Palliative care is an international concern, and there are now very few UK hospitals which don't have dedicated palliative care input. Palliative care is commonly provided in settings such as home or hospice. The hospice sector cares for over 200,000 people each year with terminal and life-limiting conditions in the UK.[1] Unfortunately, even in developed countries, specialised palliative care can often be provided only in the last weeks of life.

Many, including practitioners as well as members of the public, are concerned with the creeping trend to make a death a 'medicalised' abnormal event: 'in modern healthcare, fewer doctors and nurses have opportunity to witness normal, uncomplicated dying as their practice increasingly entangles technology with terminal care'.[2]

In 2017, it was noted that:[3]

A new Macmillan Cancer Support survey in the UK shows that although only 1% of cancer patients express a preference to die in hospital, more than a third end up there. Overall, only 20% of patients in the UK die at home, the rest dying in an institution, including hospitals, hospices and residential care.

Delirium is common in palliative care, and so merits special attention; for example, data from three North-East England hospices recently highlighted that knowledge of delirium is variable, leading to uncertainty about what constitutes delirium in hospice inpatients with subsequent difficulties in management.[4]

What is 'palliative care'?

Delirium is a major source of suffering for people receiving palliative care in hospital, and their families. Furthermore, prognosis is a key driver of clinical decision-making, and delirium is an established prognostic factor in certain settings such as advanced cancer.[5]

The World Health Organization (WHO) defines **palliative care** as:[6]

> an approach that improves the quality of life of patients and their families facing the problem associated with life-threatening illness, through the prevention and relief of suffering by means of early identification and impeccable assessment and treatment of pain and other problems, physical, psychosocial and spiritual.

Delirium under-recognition strikingly does not align with the WHO definition of palliative care, which promotes prompt assessment and preventative action to optimise patient-centred care and relief of distressing symptoms at the end of life.

Hospice UK plays a key national role in improving the quality of all palliative and end-of-life care by sharing good practice, innovative solutions and learning, not just in hospices, and equipping those professionals with the knowledge, skills and expertise needed to deliver care in any setting, to support their local communities and to work in partnership with others.[7]

A key thrust of palliative care is the promotion of dignity.

Dignity is a concept that pervades health policy, practice and biographical accounts of care. It is multifaceted and complex with various definitions in the literature, leading to difficulties in assessing the efficacy of 'dignity interventions' in practice.

How is 'palliative care' relevant to delirium?

Delirium occurs in palliative care in the context of important, life-changing illnesses, such as dementia, stroke or cancer, and can be complicated. Delirium in advanced cancer is considered a multifactorial process; a single cause of delirium can be identified for only one in three cancer patients who present a change in mental status.[8]

The prevalence of delirium among adults receiving palliative care appears similar to that among hospitalised adults with acute illness.[9] The core clinical features of delirium in palliative care, as indeed described throughout this book, are the rapid onset of disturbed attention, fluctuating levels of consciousness, cognitive impairment, psychomotor disturbance and disruption of the sleep–wake cycle.

Within palliative care, these core features can often show themselves as purposeless repetitive movements, such as plucking at bed sheets and removing clothes, accompanied by moaning and facial grimacing. Emotional changes, such as fear, anxiety and agitation, are common. Multifocal myoclonus, which may reflect opioid toxicity, renal failure or other drug-related toxicity, may be seen.

Use of the actual term 'delirium' can be infrequent in both hospital and hospice palliative care settings, and routine screening for delirium in palliative care has been low.[10] Prevalence rates of up to 88% at the end of life (last hours to weeks of life) have been reported.[11] Overall, the diagnosis of delirium is frequently missed or misdiagnosed in multiple clinical settings due to fluctuating symptoms and signs, in addition to a lack of routine cognitive screening and assessment of attention.

It is conceivable that the scope of palliative care should be broadened and provided much earlier in the disease trajectory for both malignant and non-malignant conditions, ensuring the provision of good-quality palliative and end-of-life care for all. Palliative care is applicable anywhere in a person's illness trajectory, from diagnosis to end of life, and includes bereavement support. Timing for palliative care can be inappropriately late for patients who commonly present clinical problems early in the course of disease. Palliative care is provided by specialists and generalists across various care settings to meet patient needs: specialist inpatient palliative care units, acute care with 'hospital consult teams', and community palliative care services.[12] Even among patients seen by palliative care, delirium is highly heterogeneous.[13]

The importance of palliative care delirium research

It is clear that delirium will have an increasingly significant presence in the entire remit of palliative care and thus constitutes both a service provision and a research priority. There is an interface between delirium research and palliative care research. Despite its high prevalence and incidence of delirium in palliative care settings, delirium is remarkably under-researched in the settings of palliative care.

It is not completely clear why delirium has been so relatively understudied, but a number of aspects including complexity, stability and overall phenomenology have been suggested as causes.[14] Comorbidity levels tend to increase with both age and disease progression, as do levels of troublesome symptoms, which collectively add to the challenge of assessing comprehensively delirium.

NICE has called for more research to understand the best ways of managing delirium in people at the end of their lives. This is because the current practice for relieving the distress associated with delirium often involves using medicines that can also cause sedation. In an enquiry about non-pharmacological approaches to manage delirium in patients, six themes were identified (see Box 11.1).

BOX 11.1 SIX WAYS TO HELP MANAGE DELIRIUM WITHOUT MEDICATIONS[15]

1. Orientation to time and place
2. Environmental changes
3. Familiarisation
4. Enabling autonomy
5. Soothing and distraction
6. Tactile stimulation

Diagnosing delirium in the palliative care setting

The ideal approach to making a diagnosis of delirium in palliative care would be to conduct the assessments in the traditional manner; however, a significant conflict arises in the context of the palliative care setting where the burden of assessment and investigation has to be weighed against the need for thoroughness, especially in the dying phase. The use of delirium screening tools in palliative care has been inconsistent.[16] A consensus opinion on whether screening should be done routinely and with which tool is lacking.

A recent systematic review noted that eight different screening tools vary in their feasibility, acceptability, validity, purpose, procedures, number of items and extent to which they correlated with the DSM criteria.[17]

Under-recognition of delirium in palliative care can be attributed in part to a lack of routine screening in this setting. Delirium under-recognition may be linked to a range of factors, including widely differing presentations, with fluctuating symptoms and gaps in knowledge of clinicians.[18] Although it is appropriate to omit cognitive screening in some cases – for example, where a patient is imminently dying – delirium is potentially being missed in some cases where screening would be appropriate.

Reasons given for non-completion of screening in hospice inpatient units have included descriptions of patients as 'not obviously confused' or 'alert and orientated'.[19] The hypoactive subtype of delirium is predominant in palliative care; it has a quiet, lethargic presentation that is easily mistaken for other common problems in this population, namely fatigue or depression.[20]

How is delirium managed in palliative and end-of-life care?

There could be a greater number of high-quality randomised controlled trials for delirium in palliative and end-of-life care.

It has been suggested that studies of non-pharmacological delirium interventions have frequently excluded and under-characterised people requiring palliative care, and subsequently their outcomes were infrequently reported.[21] Guidelines recommending non-pharmacological interventions as the first approach to prevent and treat delirium during advanced illness and at the end of life may not be evidence-based.[22]

The precise definition of 'end of life' has been considered elsewhere.[23]

Delirium in palliative and end-of-life contexts merits special analysis for a number of reasons. For example:

1. Iatrogenic drug causes need to be diagnosed promptly. Active de-prescribing of deliriogenic medications is a critical component of delirium management in palliative care. For example, many patients with end-stage disease may receive opioids for pain and/or dyspnoea. Opioid-induced neurotoxicity is a difficult syndrome of neuropsychiatric adverse effects that may occur with opioid therapy, and is exacerbated by a large dose, or rapid increase in opioid dose, and dehydration.

2. In patients with advanced cancer, electrolyte abnormalities including high corrected calcium levels usually cause significant problems, including delirium.

3. Effective hydration and nutrition can be significant problems.

4. Different types of delirium may have special significance. In a recent prospective cohort study, the hypoactive and mixed subtypes of delirium were found to be associated with shorter survival periods in terminally ill patients, and these associations interacted significantly with age.[24]

Effective amelioration of troublesome symptoms including delirium, pain, fatigue, difficulty in swallowing, difficulty in breathing, constipation and nausea can help a patient to have a 'good death'. Carers play a vital role in supporting the patient approaching end of life. Two arms of helping carers of people approaching end of life are intuitively desirable: support for the carer themselves and support for the carer to support the patient.

Communication about dying

Families of patients desire a more active role in care, but there are many sources of uncertainty: clarification of the known clinical status; the trajectory of the illness; the functional status prior to the episode of delirium; the desire for any further investigation; the setting of realistic goals.[25]

In the Royal College of Physicians of London/Marie Curie report *End of Life Care Audit – Dying in Hospital: National Report for England 2016*, describing all the key symptoms that could be present around the time of death, there was documented evidence that agitation/delirium existed in 72% of patients. The same audit mooted that if there is a possibility that a patient might die within days or hours, 'this possibility is recognised and communicated clearly, decisions made and actions taken in accordance with the person's needs and wishes, and these are regularly reviewed and decisions revised accordingly'.[26] Communication between physicians and dying patients about end-of-life care has been said to occur infrequently; when it does occur, studies suggest that there are significant deficiencies in the quality of this communication.[27]

There are also, arguably, significant gaps in knowledge and communications skills of new-entrant doctors around the legal, ethical and practical aspects of end-of-life care. A recent study[28] advised that further training may be required to prepare junior doctors for patient death and end-of-life care. Junior doctors require support when dealing with distressing clinical situations. Nurses also play an important role in helping families understand the dying process by communicating clear, direct and consistent patient information using easily understood language.

'Terminal delirium' and the 'reversibility' of delirium

Regardless of whether delirium is ultimately preventable or reversible for the individual patient, optimal person-centred palliative care is possible. Deciding if the delirium is reversible or irreversible alone can be an ethical dilemma as valuable time may be wasted in a futile efforts during the investigation and diagnosis, while potentially leaving a patient suffering.

Reversible delirium and irreversible delirium often share a very similar clinical presentation; they may be indistinguishable until basic clinical (laboratory and sometimes radiological) investigations are completed. In palliative care, evidence suggests that approximately 50% of delirium episodes can be reversed,[29] especially those precipitated by medications, infection and electrolyte abnormalities.

A 'terminal delirium' occurs in the last days and hours of life, often as a result of end-stage multisystem organ failure and other irreversible factors. Clinical features of a terminal delirium, such as 'moaning, groaning, and facial grimacing',[30] might be interpreted as pain and this is often a source of distress to families and carers. This term is, however, not without some controversy in the field, because delirium can still be reversible in palliative care, and interventions promoting good health should be encouraged where realistic.

Palliative sedation

The goal of **palliative sedation** is to relieve pain and suffering, never to shorten life. According to the European Association for Palliative Care (EAPC), it is defined as 'the monitored use of medications intended to induce a state of decreased or absent awareness in order to relieve the burden of otherwise intractable suffering'.[31] Palliative sedation is used for refractory symptoms that many advanced cancer and non-cancer patients experience in the last days of life and which cannot be controlled even by the best palliative therapies otherwise.

In spite of aggressive palliative measures, symptom management can sometimes become challenging at end of life. Systematic reviews of research involving the use of palliative sedation indicate that this intervention does not shorten patients' survival.[32]

Benzodiazepines remain a mainstay of treatment of palliative sedation. Midazolam is widely used because it has a fast onset but also a short half-life, which allows rapid titration, and may be given intravenously or subcutaneously. Midazolam is one of three most frequently administered drugs in palliative medicine, the others being morphine and haloperidol.[33]

Delirium and agitation

Agitation is often a symptom of delirium, but some patients can become agitated without having delirium; agitation might be due to symptoms such as pain or breathlessness.[34] Delirium and agitation are frequent occurrences in patients in general and, more often, near the end of life as is common in the palliative care setting. However, there is some doubt about the best regimens to control the different aspects of care that patients with delirium need.

Haloperidol is used alone for the control of agitation in different settings. However, the issues are complex; for example, in a recent review, the use of haloperidol alone was considered unethical for psychosis-induced aggression where additional drugs are available to offset the adverse effects.[35]

Benzodiazepines alone do not seem to be adequate for the control of agitation either, and even might be a risk factor[36] for delirium development, unless the cause is alcohol or benzodiazepines withdrawal.

There is a need to identify those factors contributing to communication capacity impairment and agitated delirium. High-dose opioid requirement has been identified as a significant determinant of impaired communication capacity.[37]

Endnotes

1   Hospice UK (2019) 'Facts and figures: About hospice care.' Accessed on 2/12/2019 at www.hospiceuk. org/about-hospice-care/media-centre/facts-and-figures.

2   Mannix, K. (2017) *With the End in Mind: How to Live and Die Well*. London: William Collins.

3   Srivastava, R. (2017) 'Dying at home might sound preferable. But I've seen the reality.' *The Guardian*, 1 May. Accessed on 2/12/2019 at www.theguardian.com/commentisfree/2017/may/01/dying-at-home-terminally-ill-hospital.

4   Waterfield, K., Kiltie, R., Pickard, J., Karandikhar, U. *et al.* (2017) 'P-28 Staff experiences of delirium in the hospice setting.' *BMJ Supportive and Palliative Care 7*, 1. Accessed on 2/12/2019 at https://spcare. bmj.com/content/7/Suppl_1/A10.2.

5   Hui, D. (2015) 'Prognostication of survival in patients with advanced cancer: Predicting the unpredictable.' *Cancer Control 22*, 4, 489–497. Accessed on 2/12/2019 at www.ncbi.nlm.nih.gov/pubmed/26678976.

6   World Health Organization (2019) 'WHO Definition of Palliative Care.' Accessed on 2/12/2019 at www.who.int/cancer/palliative/definition/en.

7   Hospice UK (2019) 'What we do.' Accessed on 2/12/2019 at www.hospiceuk.org/about-us/what-we-do.

8   Centeno, C., Sanz, A. and Bruera, E. (2004) 'Delirium in advanced cancer patients.' *Palliative Medicine 18*, 3, 184–194. Accessed on 2/12/2019 at www.ncbi.nlm.nih.gov/pubmed/15198131.

9   National Institute for Health Research (2018) 'Delirium is common among adults receiving palliative care and could be better recognised.' Accessed on 2/12/2019 at https://discover.dc.nihr.ac.uk/content/ signal-000677/delirium-recognition-in-palliative-care.

10   Boland, J.W., Lawlor, P.G. and Bush, S.H. (2019) 'Delirium: Non-pharmacological and pharmacological management.' *BMJ Supportive and Palliative Care*. doi: 10.1136/bmjspcare-2019-001966. Accessed on 2/12/2019 at https://spcare.bmj.com/content/early/2019/07/30/bmjspcare-2019-001966.abstract.

11   National Institute for Health Research (2018) 'Delirium is common among adults receiving palliative care and could be better recognised.' Accessed on 2/12/2019 at https://discover.dc.nihr.ac.uk/content/ signal-000677/delirium-recognition-in-palliative-care.

12   Bush, S.H., Tierney, S. and Lawlor, P.G. (2017) 'Clinical assessment and management of delirium in the palliative care setting.' *Drugs 77*, 15, 1623–1643. Accessed on 2/12/2019 at www.ncbi.nlm.nih.gov/pmc/ articles/PMC5613058.

13   Hui, D. (2019) 'Delirium in the palliative care setting: "Sorting" out the confusion.' *Palliative Medicine*. Accessed on 2/12/2019 at https://journals.sagepub.com/doi/10.1177/0269216319861896.

14   Lawlor, P.G., Davis, D.H.J., Ansari, M., Hosie, A. *et al.* (2014) 'An analytical framework for delirium research in palliative care settings: Integrated epidemiologic, clinician-researcher, and knowledge user perspectives.' *Journal of Pain and Symptom Management 48*, 2, 159–175. Accessed on 2/12/2019 at www. ncbi.nlm.nih.gov/pmc/articles/PMC4128755/

15 Marie Curie (2018) 'Improving support for people with delirium and their carers.' Accessed on 2/12/2019 at www.mariecurie.org.uk/blog/support-for-people-with-delirium/183059

16 Porteous, A., Dewhurst, F., Grogan, E., Lowery, L. et al. 'How common is delirium in palliative care inpatient units and what is the outcome for these patients?' BMJ Supportive and Palliative Care 4, A61. Accessed on 2/12/2019 at https://spcare.bmj.com/content/4/Suppl_1/A61.3.

17 Porteous, A., Dewhurst, F., Gray, W.K., Coulter, P. et al. (2016) 'Screening for delirium in specialist palliative care inpatient units: Perceptions and outcomes.' International Journal of Palliative Nursing 22, 9, 444–447. Accessed on 2/12/2019 at www.ncbi.nlm.nih.gov/pubmed/27666305.

18 Hosie, A., Lobb, E., Agar, M., Davidson, P.M. and Phillips, J. (2014) 'Identifying the barriers and enablers to palliative care nurses' recognition and assessment of delirium symptoms: A qualitative study.' Journal of Pain and Symptom Management 48, 5, 815–830. Accessed on 2/12/2019 at www.ncbi.nlm.nih.gov/pubmed/24726761.

19 Smith, J. and Adcock, L. (2011) 'The recognition of delirium in hospice inpatient units.' Palliative Medicine 26, 3, 283–285. Accessed on 2/12/2019 at https://journals.sagepub.com/doi/full/10.1177/0269216311400932.

20 de Wolf-Linder, S., Dawkins, M., Wicks, F., Pask, S. et al. (2019) 'Which outcome domains are important in palliative care and when? An international expert consensus workshop, using the nominal group technique.' Palliative Medicine 33, 8, 1058–1068. Accessed on 2/12/2019 at https://journals.sagepub.com/doi/full/10.1177/0269216319854154.

21 Hosie, A., Siddiqi, N., Featherstone, I., Johnson, M. et al. (2019) 'Inclusion, characteristics and outcomes of people requiring palliative care in studies of non-pharmacological interventions for delirium.' Palliative Medicine 33, 8, 878–899. Accessed on 2/12/2019 at https://journals.sagepub.com/doi/full/10.1177/0269216319853487.

22 Hosie, A., Siddiqi, N., Featherstone, I., Johnson, M. et al. (2019) 'Inclusion, characteristics and outcomes of people requiring palliative care in studies of non-pharmacological interventions for delirium.' Palliative Medicine 33, 8, 878–899. Accessed on 2/12/2019 at https://journals.sagepub.com/doi/full/10.1177/0269216319853487.

23 Hui, D., Nooruddin, Z., Didwaniya, N., Dev, R. et al. (2013) 'Concepts and definitions for "actively dying", "end of life", "terminally ill", "terminal care", and "transition of care": A systematic review.' Journal of Pain and Symptom Management 47, 1, 77–89. Accessed on 2/12/2019 at www.ncbi.nlm.nih.gov/pmc/articles/PMC3870193.

24 Kim, S.Y., Kim, S.W., Kim, J.M. and Shin, I.S. (2015) 'Differential associations between delirium and mortality according to delirium subtype and age: A prospective cohort study.' Psychosomatic Medicine 77, 8, 903–910. Accessed on 2/12/2019 at www.ncbi.nlm.nih.gov/pubmed/26397939.

25 Bush, S.H., Tierney, S. and Lawlor, P.G. (2017) 'Clinical assessment and management of delirium in the palliative care setting.' Drugs 77, 15, 1623–1643. Accessed on 2/12/2019 at www.ncbi.nlm.nih.gov/pmc/articles/PMC5613058.

26 Royal College of Physicians (2015) End of Life Care Audit: Dying in Hospital. Accessed on 2/12/2019 at www.rcplondon.ac.uk/projects/end-life-care-audit-dying-hospital.

27 Wenrich, M.D., Curtis, J.R. and Shannon, S.E., (2001) 'Communicating with dying patients within the spectrum of medical care from terminal diagnosis to death.' JAMA Internal Medicine 161, 6, 868–874. Accessed on 2/12/2019 at https://jamanetwork.com/journals/jamainternalmedicine/fullarticle/647723.

28 Linane, H., Connolly, F., McVicker, L., Beatty, S. et al. (2019) 'Disturbing and distressing: A mixed methods study on the psychological impact of end of life care on junior doctors.' Irish Journal of Medical Science 188, 2, 633–639. Accessed on 2/12/2019 at https://link.springer.com/article/10.1007/s11845-018-1885-z.

29 Bush, S.H., Tierney, S. and Lawlor, P.G. (2017) 'Clinical assessment and management of delirium in the palliative care setting.' Drugs 77, 15, 1623–1643. Accessed on 2/12/2019 at www.ncbi.nlm.nih.gov/pmc/articles/PMC5613058.

30 Bush, S.H., Leonard, M.M., Agar, M., Spiller, J.A. et al. (2014) 'End-of-life delirium: Issues regarding recognition, optimal management, and the role of sedation in the dying phase.' Journal of Pain and Symptom Management 48, 2, 215–230. Accessed on 2/12/2019 at www.jpsmjournal.com/article/S0885-3924(14)00288-7/fulltext.

31 Schur, S., Weixler, D., Gabl, C., Kreye, G. et al. (2016) 'Sedation at the end of life – a nation-wide study in palliative care in Austria.' BMC Palliative Care 15, 50. Accessed on 2/12/2019 at www.ncbi.nlm.nih.gov/pmc/articles/PMC4868021.

32   Twycross, R. (2019) 'Reflections on palliative sedation.' *Palliative Care 12*, 1178224218823511. Accessed on 2/12/2019 at www.ncbi.nlm.nih.gov/pmc/articles/PMC635016.

33   Masman, A.D., van Dijk, M., Tibboel, D., Baar, F.P.M. and Mathôt, R.A.A., (2015) 'Medication use during end-of-life care in a palliative care centre.' *International Journal of Clinical Pharmacy 37*, 5, 767–775. Accessed on 2/12/2019 at www.ncbi.nlm.nih.gov/pmc/articles/PMC4594093.

34   Marie Curie (2019) 'Delirium.' Accessed on 2/12/2019 at www.mariecurie.org.uk/professionals/palliative-care-knowledge-zone/symptom-control/delirium.

35   *Evidence-Based Mental Health* (2013) 'Review: Limited evidence on effects of haloperidol alone for rapid tranquillisation in psychosis-induced aggression.' *Evidence-Based Mental Health 16*, 47. Accessed on 2/12/2019 at https://ebmh.bmj.com/content/16/2/47.

36   Stern, T.A., Celano, C.M., Gross, A.F. and Huffman, J.C. (2010) 'The assessment and management of agitation and delirium in the general hospital.' *Primary Care Companion to the Journal of Clinical Psychiatry 12*, 1, PCC.09r00938. Accessed on 2/12/2019 at www.ncbi.nlm.nih.gov/pmc/articles/PMC2882819.

37   Morita, T., Tei, Y. and Inouye, S. (2003) 'Impaired communication capacity and agitated delirium in the final week of terminally ill cancer patients: Prevalence and identification of research focus.' *Journal of Pain and Symptom Management 26*, 3, 827–834. Accessed on 2/12/2019 at www.sciencedirect.com/science/article/pii/S0885392403002872.

12

Quality improvement and evidence-based medicine

LEARNING OBJECTIVES

Resistance to change is common, but improving delirium care is an important challenge. There are genuine lessons to be learned about how to assess and share good practice. This chapter will give an account of some of the tools routinely used in quality improvement, such as audit cycles, PDSA (Plan, Do, Study, Act) and systematic reviews, but will also consider wider and significant issues including 'buy in' from leadership or patients/carers.

Introduction

The responsibility of providing high-quality care, from delirium screening to diagnosis to treatment, is the 'business' of every member of the multidisciplinary team, and therefore a multi-pronged strategy is needed.

Patients with delirium often receive suboptimal care, including in acute hospitals. Experience gained from quality improvement programmes in a number of jurisdictions shows that progress can be made. Identifying the gaps between desired and actual practice should be the starting point for all interventions.

Within healthcare, there is no universally accepted definition of '**quality**'. However, the following definition from the US Institute of Medicine is often used:[1]

> [Quality is] the degree to which health services for individuals and populations increase the likelihood of desired health outcomes and are consistent with current professional knowledge.

Many healthcare institutions are tasked with improving delirium care.

Key skills for anyone involved are: listen, and then build up trust. Those working in healthcare are aware of the considerable gap between what we know from research and what is done in clinical practice.

You might have read aspects in this book that are unrecognisable in your organisation's clinical practise. The problem addressed by the **quality improvement** (QI) approach might conceivably be described as the 'knowing–doing' gap: we know individually and collectively what to do, but fail to do it or fail to implement any improvement.

Barriers at each of various organisational levels might contribute to the shortcomings in fully reaching **SMART** (Specific, Measurable, Achievable, Realistic and Timely) aims in quality improvement.[2] 'Grounded theory' has been adopted as a research method to identify the practice gaps in relation to managing the patient with delirium.[3] These gaps are said to be determined by factors operating at individual, team and organisational levels.

Evidence-based medicine (EBM) and QI have overall similar goals but different priorities. There has been a marked increase in activity in research into delirium neuroscience. EBM has focused more on performing actions informed by the best available evidence from our clinical knowledge base, whereas QI has focused more on making sure that intended actions are done efficiently and reliably.

Sources of user information

User involvement acts as an important driving force for innovation. Learning may not be possible without a notion of **'agency'**, or a reframing of the process by which leaders lead change.

The concerns of users can be identified from various sources, including:

- comments or letters of complaints

- 'friends and family test'

- reports in the media

- regulators' reports

- critical incident reports

- individual patients' stories or feedback from focus groups

- direct observation of care

- direct conversations.

Peers understand and appreciate the complexities of quality improvement in healthcare. Collaboration can support innovation and progress, and reduces barriers to change. Quality improvement initiatives can be reviewed and piloted across regional and national clinical and academic networks which can be used for 'scaling up' local initiatives. Patient collaboration can encourage benefits through self-management and self-care, ultimately improving the overall quality of care received.

Barriers to quality improvement overall

With respect to improving care in the foreseeable future and translating better understandings into practice, formidable challenges exist. These include:

- practical difficulties in undertaking delirium research
- the fluctuating nature of delirium
- problems in generalising findings
- an absence of an agreed, structured approach to treatment
- cultural barriers to delirium being perceived as 'important'
- diverse 'causes' of delirium
- recognising commonalities and differences across different care settings
- the underlying cognitive status or comorbidities of patients participating in research.

Contexts of healthcare quality improvement
The local context

Your organisation is very likely to have its own transformation programme focusing on key local priorities. Some of the other priorities are relevant to delirium prevention, including a focus on sepsis or pressure ulcers.

A healthy attitude to using all feedback is helpful. Look at recent adverse events or complaints and review positive feedback from patients. Consider holding 'brainstorming' sessions to engage all members of the team active in an improvement process, emphasising that the improvement will be important and relevant to them.

Linking in with the clinical governance mechanisms and quality improvement teams will help align your work to these wider organisational goals which is helpful for senior management and leadership.

A wider context

BMJ Quality Improvement Reports[4] is an important resource because it provides a fully searchable open-access repository of quality improvement projects. Twitter, blogposts and videos might also be useful. There are many patient stories which provoke ideas on change and can provide a powerful tool for engaging people with your project.

The National Institute for Clinical and Healthcare Excellence (NICE) in the UK publishes Quality Standards for structures, process and outcomes across different clinical areas which can be used for project topics.

Teamwork

Many healthcare organisations have used multidisciplinary teams as a mechanism for bringing about improvements in quality. '**Team-building efforts**' can be essential to address interpersonal conflicts.

Teamwork is dependent on excellent communication and a focus on identifying and resolving any conflicts. It also needs genuine respect for different perspectives, and relies on a genuine commitment to learning and improving. The use of teams for quality improvement goes back to the 1930s and the work of industrial quality experts such as Joseph Juran.

Leadership and culture

Engaging frontline clinical staff is crucial for any QI programme, but in reality it can be challenging. Many senior clinicians will be keen to improve the quality of the service they offer, and will have done so through various methods already. However, they may be unfamiliar with QI approaches.

'**Communities of practice**' may encourage a culture of shared learning and participative leadership, which is particularly helpful as hierarchical leadership can even be obstructive for change. The culture must encourage staff to be open, to test new ideas and to learn from mistakes rather than to blame. The leadership has to strike the right balance between supporting staff, allowing autonomy within boundaries and excellent accountability.

QI leaders have a key role in helping their teams to work through improvement 'failures' and to promote adoption of 'successes'. '**Champions**' might be local or external opinion leaders who are seen by others as trustworthy and authentically passionate about the 'cause', and who can persuade others to implement evidence-based practice or quality improvement. The identification of barriers and facilitators is important to the work of the champion.

Change

Organisational change can substantially erode team members' sense of freedom and ability to contribute.[5] All stakeholders need to know that they are valued. The implementation of a new intervention or initiative is often met with resistance to change.

Change is not a goal in itself.

The case for a change by a social movement of various people wishing to put delirium care into a more caring space is overwhelming:

> Social movements recognise the power of disrupting the status quo and doing things differently. They often use loose and dynamic networks to encourage many different approaches simultaneously to raise their profile and address the problems they fight for. Especially in the early stages of a movement, creating an environment of experimentation, where any person or group can try out new ideas and tactics, utilising their unique strengths and skills, can be critical for success.[6]

Transformational change is defined as the 'emergence of an entirely new state, prompted by a shift in what is considered possible or necessary, which results in a profoundly different structure, culture or level of performance.'[7] It is fundamentally different from a slight incremental improvement. The vision and need for transformational change tends to concern a bold vision and values of stakeholders.

Change invariably provokes a range of emotions in people: some are sceptical of the need for it or resist it on principle, resulting in conflict. Usually, the key factor behind a successful introduction of any change is the **ownership and control** of the introduction by the staff that had to drive to deliver the process. There is an old adage: 'People don't mind change as much as they mind being changed.'

The vision and need for change must be translated into key themes that all people can understand and that they can feel passionate about. '**Change packages**' are devised by a group of stakeholders to define the required quality improvements, to identify the group of patients to be affected the most, and to establish specific quantitative measures to determine whether or not the changes led to a real improvement.

To minimise this resistance to change, a few strategies might be useful:

* discovering stakeholders' attitudes about a possible need for improvement

* educating stakeholders about the impact of bad delirium care

- addressing any operational impact on conducting a QI project
- providing useful feedback about the progress of the QI project
- a willingness to 'celebrate change'.

Implementing change through checklists

A **checklist** is an 'algorithmic listing of actions to be performed in a given clinical setting, the goal being to ensure that no step will be forgotten'.[8] Checklists have been widely discussed elsewhere.[9]

Large-scale implementations of checklists with conflicting outcomes suggest that these tools are not as simple or effective as hoped. Checklists might improve a culture of teamwork by empowering staff to speak up about potential safety matters, but they might be viewed by some staff as rather 'robotic'.

There are reasons for varying outcomes in the use of checklists:

- wider cultural and organisational change efforts are required, not just the checklist itself
- the roles of individual team members in implementing the checklist need to be clarified
- the contribution of leadership
- training of individuals implementing checklists.

Patient and carer involvement

A study by the Health Foundation indicates that 'interpersonal behaviours', focusing on relationships between people in the system, are crucial to understand.[10] Developing, maintaining and using strategic alliances are at the heart of quality improvement, and patients, carers and the wider public have a significant role to play in driving the case for QI. Patients may define quality differently from clinicians and managers. What they view as the 'problem' or value within a system may be surprising to practitioners and professionals.

Leaders need to question how patient involvement is being embedded in their organisations' QI programmes. The involvement of patients in healthcare QI can take many forms, such as:

- patient representation at organisational quality committees and in research panels

- shadowing the patient journey to identify quality gaps and shortfalls
- patient-led assessment of the healthcare environment
- completion of 'patient satisfaction surveys'
- review of content and style of patient information materials
- patient networking to share self-care strategies
- analysis of patient complaints, concerns and claims
- patient involvement in QI focus groups.

Equity and equality considerations

The World Health Organization defines **equity** as the absence of avoidable, unfair or remediable differences among groups of people.[11] Improving quality is about making healthcare safe, efficient, effective, patient-centred, timely and equitable. Health equity is all about fairness and justice, and implies that everyone should have an equal opportunity to achieve the best delirium care.

Benchmarking

Benchmarking is the process of comparing one's performance to that of others.

The formal practice of benchmarking is a relatively recent innovation in the quality management sciences, having been developed in the 1980s at Xerox. An organisation performing less well may seek the advice of one performing well.

In a sense, 'best practices' do not exist, as we can always strive to do better.

Best-practice guidelines for delirium detection and management are based on consensus, as well as high-level evidence for delirium management. They include:

- NICE (National Institute for Health and Care Excellence): 'Delirium: prevention, diagnosis and management', clinical guideline [CG103] (2010), www.nice.org.uk/guidance/cg103.

- SIGN (Scottish Intercollegiate Guidelines Network): 'Risk reduction and management of delirium' (SIGN 157, 2019), www.sign.ac.uk/sign-157-delirium.html.

Further important guidelines include:

- Australian Commission on Safety and Quality in Healthcare: 'Delirium Clinical Care Standard' (2017), www.safetyandquality. gov.au/our-work/clinical-care-standards/delirium-clinical-care-standard.

- American Geriatrics Society Clinical Practice Guidelines for Post-operative Delirium in Older Adults (2014), https://geriatrics careonline. org/ProductAbstract/american-geriatrics-society-clinical-practice-guideline-for-postoperative-delirium-in-older-adults/CL018.

Davis, Searle and Tsui write:[12]

The publication of the Scottish Intercollegiate Guidelines Network (SIGN) guideline on delirium is a state-of-the-art synthesis of the field. It consolidates previous work and guidelines, not least the pivotal publication of NICECG103, yet offers new recommendations, particularly around detection and a more explicit focus on communication and follow-up.

They further comment:

The SIGN guidelines are published at a time when interest in, and concern for, older frail people is high; the individual and societal impact of health problems in ageing is apparent to all. If delirium is a measure of the degree to which we as healthcare professionals practice with compassion, then the imperative will be to make continued headway on improving delirium care in all respects. These guidelines on delirium are an important component of that future.

Nurses and delirium

To promote participation and 'buy in', QI leaders need to create a connection, build bridges and communicate the vision.

Nurses, who spend more time at the bedside than physicians, play a crucial role in the recognition of delirium. In terms of delirium recognition and screening, nurses occupy a uniquely strategic position in inpatient care; their 24-hour level of patient contact affords an ideal opportunity to observe and record the fluctuating feature of delirium symptoms. They are better able to observe fluctuations in attention, level of consciousness and cognitive functioning. It is desirable to coordinate care to achieve meaningful communication according to changes in consciousness levels during the day.

Engaging families is also a premium consideration. Family members' distress might be reduced by providing the resources for them to participate in caregiving. They can participate by assisting with reorientation, communication and aspects of personal care.

Self-evaluation

Using self-evaluation for quality improvement, rather than undertaking evaluation only in response to external scrutiny, offers a structured way to encourage local dissemination of outcomes and impacts, and to inspire greater local ownership of issues and design of more effective solutions.

Improvement cycles and 'PDSA'

PDSA has its origins in the work of Schewart and Deming.[13]

A first step in implementing a clinical practice guideline is to gain an understanding of current clinical practice.

The 'Model for Improvement' from the Associates in Process Improvement asks three questions:[14]

- What are we trying to accomplish?

- How will we know change is an improvement?

- What changes can we make that will result in the improvements that we seek?

Audit tools should be comprehensive but not time-consuming to use.

The **plan, do study, act (PDSA)** quality improvement methodology uses a four-step approach to implementing changes to improve quality of care. The method is widely used in healthcare improvement; however, there is little overarching evaluation of how the method is applied.

The four stages mirror the scientific method of formulating a hypothesis, collecting data to test this hypothesis, analysing and interpreting the results, and making inferences to iterate the hypothesis.

The pragmatic principles of PDSA cycles promote the use of a small-scale, iterative approach to test interventions, to enable a rapid assessment and provide flexibility to adapt the change according to feedback to ensure that fit-for-purpose solutions are developed. Sharing the results, whatever they are, is ultimately important.

Possible other targets for auditing are shown in Box 12.1.

BOX 12.1 POSSIBLE TOPICS FOR AN AUDIT IN DELIRIUM

The percentage of:

- at-risk patients assessed for delirium
- patients in a critical care environment assessed for delirium
- patients in a care home who develop delirium
- patients with confirmed delirium who are recorded and coded with delirium, and the diagnosis is included in discharge summaries to the GP
- patients with delirium who are then identified for the first time as having a background cognitive impairment
- patients who have medication reviews
- patients experiencing delirium in hospital who are followed up by the primary care team.

The basic 'nuts and bolts' of the PDSA approach are shown in Box 12.2.

BOX 12.2 PDSA

Plan: Decide when, how and where the plan will be implemented. Specific objectives as well as predictions of outcome should be stated in this phase.

Do: Carry out the plan and document relevant data that identify successes, problems or unexpected outcomes.

Study: Evaluate the documented data to determine if the plan is working. Results are compared to those predicted. You can demonstrate improvement with a relatively small number of data points.

Act: The intervention being tested is adopted, adapted or rejected.

Starting with small-scale tests provides users with freedom to act and learn, minimising risk to patients, the organisation and resources required, and providing the opportunity to build evidence for change and engage stakeholders as confidence in the intervention increases.

Systematic reviews and meta-analysis

Systematic reviews and meta-analyses are increasingly common. Failure of the timely use of systematic reviews and meta-analysis might lead to unnecessary harm in patient care.

A good systematic review will not only identify the published and unpublished literature on a specific question, but summarise the findings, critically evaluate the included studies and make recommendations about future research. Systematic reviews ideally should avoid bias and should be reproducible.

Meta-analysis uses optimum techniques to provide pooled estimates of association, such as treatment effects.

A well-conducted **randomised controlled trial (RCT)** is considered the highest form of evidence for assessing the effect of interventions. In an RCT, one group is allocated to receive an intervention and the other receive a control.

Observational studies include **cohort** and **case–control** designs, and can all be described as non-randomised.

Observational studies can provide evidence of associations between factors, but they cannot prove that an observed relationship is causative.

A cohort study is simply a set of individuals who share some characteristic and who are followed up over time. Case–control studies retrospectively compare individuals with a disease ('cases') with matched 'controls' without that disease, to understand which factors are associated with the development of the disease.

Criticising a QI initiative

An important part of carrying out a QI project is enabling others to learn from your experiences. You will be invited to contemplate the lessons you learned from the project and its limitations. Reflecting on what you've learned from your QI study will help to avoid unnecessary duplication from other investigators elsewhere, and will also help others to learn from your concerns.

- Comment on the strengths of the project. What's 'new'?

- Describe any problems you faced and how you overcame these. If you were to undertake this project again, what would you do differently?

- Reflect on your project's limitations. Are there any limits on generalisability due to where the study took place?

- Describe whether chance bias, or confounding have affected your results?

- Is the sample size too small?

Methodological concerns
Bias
Bias is an incorrect estimation of the association – for example, between exposure and outcome – due to a systematic error. Bias can be a serious threat to valid inference but too vigorous an attack on bias can have unanticipated perverse effects.

Inclusion/exclusion criteria
Are the people included similar to what tends to happen in everyday clinical practice? For example, are people appropriately excluded on the basis of age or comorbidities that are actually quite common in the group defined?

Clinical audit
Clinical audit is a quality improvement process with the aim of improving patient care and outcomes through systematic review of care against explicit criteria and the implementation and communication of changes.

Aspects of the structure, processes and outcomes of care are selected and systematically evaluated against explicit criteria. An audit cycle could be used, for example, to reassess if a hospital has improved its assessment of delirium diagnosis, prevention and management after raising awareness of delirium through an education, training and dissemination of delirium care bundle throughout a hospital trust.[15]

The main stages of the clinical audit process are shown in Box 12.3.

BOX 12.3 AUDIT CYCLE

Select a topic.

A clear sense of purpose must be established.

↓

Agreeing standards of best practice (audit criteria).

Process criteria refer to the actions and decisions taken by practitioners together with users.

Outcome criteria are typically measures of the response to an intervention, e.g. level of knowledge and satisfaction.

↓

Collect data appropriately (qualitatively and/or quantitatively).

↓

Analyse data against standards using the most appropriate methods.

↓

Feed back results.

Discuss possible changes.

↓

Implement and communicate agreed changes.

↓

Re-audit.

↓

Feed back the re-audit results.

↓

Discuss whether practice has actually improved.

This iterative process is called the '**audit cycle**'.

At a local level, clinical audit links into both clinical effectiveness and clinical governance.

Spread and uptake of 'products of change'

Having implemented your intervention locally, it is important to consider how you intervention will be rolled out. This has practical considerations.

Some points to consider are:

- Which teams or departments are you going to target?

- Which groups of employees within these are key – for example, clinical specialist nurses, HCAs or ward managers?

- How are you are going to let staff know about the intervention?

- How will you encourage adopters to engage?

- How will you get feedback?

In healthcare services research, one may utilise Rogers'[16] extensively used model, which pictures the adoption of an innovation as a **five-stage process**:

1. Basic knowledge about the intervention.

2. The formation of favourable or unfavourable attitudes towards the innovation.

3. The 'actors' make a decision to adopt or reject the innovation.

4. 'Actors' must evaluate the new product as a positive contribution to everyday life or work environment.

5. The practical consequences of applying the intervention have a strong influence on the ultimate adoption of the intervention.

Criticisms can be made of the concept of 'fixed adopter characteristics' of an innovation: in reality, decisions about adopting complex innovations are influenced to a large extent by a contextual judgement.

Endnotes

1   Institute of Medicine (1990) *Crossing the Quality Chasm: A New Health System for the 21st Century.* Washington, DC: National Academy Press, p.244.

2   Chartered Management Institute (2011) 'Setting SMART Objectives Checklist.' Accessed on 2/12/2019 at www.managers.org.uk/~/media/Files/Campus%20CMI/Checklists%20PDP/Setting%20SMART%20 objectives.ashx.

3   Teodorczuk, A., Mukaetova-Ladinska, E., Corbett, S. and Welfare, M. (2015) 'Deconstructing dementia and delirium hospital practice: Using cultural historical activity theory to inform education approaches.' *Advances in Health Sciences Education: Theory and Practice 20,* 3, 745–764. Accessed on 2/12/2019 at www.ncbi.nlm.nih.gov/pubmed/25354660.

4   See https://bmjopenquality.bmj.com//?gclid=CjwKCAjw36DpBRAYEiwAmVVDMEgLccfSVfxzSkY wZova5uggH7DovPTzOIH0mzW4ee9 xckV3nNRQEhoCOsAQAvD_BwE.

5   NHS (2010) *The Handbook of Quality and Service Improvement Tools.* Accessed on 2/12/2019 at https:// webarchive.nationalarchives.gov.uk/20160805121829/http:/www.nhsiq.nhs.uk/media/2760650/the_ handbook_of_quality_and_service_improvement_tools_2010.pdf.

6   del Castillo, J., Nicholas, L., Nye, R. and Khan, H. (2017) 'We change the world: What can we learn from global social movements for health?' *Nesta.* Accessed on 2/12/2019 at https://media.nesta.org.uk/ documents/we_change_the_world_report.pdf, p.11.

7   Dougall, D., Lewis, M. and Ross, S. (2018) *Transformational Change in Health and Care: Reports from the Field.* The King's Fund. Accessed on 2/12/2019 at www.kingsfund.org.uk/publications/transformational-change-health-care.

8   Patient Safety Network (2019) 'Patient Safety Primer: Checklists.' Accessed on 2/12/2019 at https://psnet. ahrq.gov/primer/checklists

9   Catchpole, K. and Russ, S. (2015) 'The problem with checklists.' *BMJ Quality and Safety 24,* 9. Accessed on 2/12/2019 at https://qualitysafety.bmj.com/content/24/9/545.

10 The Health Foundation (2011) 'Evidence: What's leadership got to do with it? Exploring links between quality improvement and leadership in the NHS. Accessed on 2/12/2019 at www.health.org.uk/sites/ default/files/WhatsLeadershipGotToDoWithIt.pdf.

11 World Health Organization (n.d.) 'Equity.' Accessed on 2/12/2019 at www.who.int/healthsystems/topics/ equity/en.

12 Davis, D., Searle, S.D. and Tsui, A. (2019) 'The Scottish Intercollegiate Guidelines Network: Risk reduction and management of delirium.' *Age and Ageing 48,* 4, 485–488. Accessed on 2/12/2019 at www. ncbi.nlm.nih.gov/pubmed/30927352, pp.2, 3.

13 Moen, R. (2009) 'Foundation and history of the PDSA Cycle.' Accessed on 2/12/2019 at https://deming. org/uploads/paper/PDSA_History_Ron_Moen.pdf.

14 Institute for Healthcare Improvement (2019) 'How to improve.' Accessed on 2/12/2019 at www.ihi.org/ resources/Pages/HowtoImprove/default.aspx.

15 Khan, W. (2019) 'An audit cycle demonstrating improvement in delirium diagnosis, prevention and management (NICE guideline) at a district general hospital.' *Future Healthcare Journal 6,* suppl.1, 14. Accessed on 2/12/2019 at www.ncbi.nlm.nih.gov/pubmed/31363539.

16 NSW Agency for Clinical Innovation (2015) 'Change Management Theories and Models – Everett Rogers.' Accessed on 16/12/2019 at www.aci.health.nsw.gov.au/__data/assets/pdf_file/0010/298756/ Change_Management_Theories_and_Models_Everett_Rogers.pdf.

13

Educational initiatives

LEARNING OBJECTIVES

In this final chapter, you will be encouraged to think about how you might inspire others to learn about delirium, provide better care for patients with delirium, and to take further your continuous professional education and service improvement in delirium. Much progress has been made in educational initiatives in recent years, ranging from traditional grand rounds to e-learning and even Twitter. You can be a part of that social movement.

Raising awareness of delirium

Educational innovations in delirium should be offered for all healthcare professionals at pre- and post-qualifying levels, and, where possible, should be freely accessible. In order to overcome organisational barriers to good practice, communicating with senior healthcare managers to situate delirium on the management agenda is possibly an important 'driver for change'.

Educational initiatives need to be embedded in any quality improvement experience. Delirium education is not a 'big bang event', but an iterative process. The awareness and detection of delirium has been shown to improve significantly with a targeted education of healthcare professionals and the implementation of focused care pathways.

A need to place delirium on an equal footing to other medical disorders is important. There needs to be greater prioritisation of delirium both in the curriculum and as a service consideration.

Strategies might include the use of widespread patient information leaflets explaining in lay language the importance of delirium, but this may be insufficient in itself to bring about a sea change in attitudes. Videos involving carers and patients could be developed and used as teaching tools to understand the patient experience.

Public lectures and awareness events (such as a 'Delirium Fair') could help promote an understanding of the reasons why patients with delirium do so badly in general hospitals. In contrast to other common illnesses in later life, there currently exist no dedicated patient groups (e.g. Alzheimer's Society in the UK) which could raise the profile and help educate the public and ultimately change attitudes. Finally, there is a need for responsibly ensuring that all care settings are represented in educational initiatives – including care homes.

The importance of delirium education

Education is at the heart of driving up standards of care; it would be great if educational interventions on delirium improve recognition of the condition, reduce its severity and even reduce length of hospital stay.

Educational interventions around delirium diagnosis and treatment also have the capacity to improve confidence around delirium assessment as well as knowledge of delirium care. Incorporating delirium prevention into routine clinical practice continues to be challenging, but an education programme focused on 'knowing, meaning and doing', consisting of a brief online course, case discussions with experts and a high-fidelity simulation, might be effective.[1] Good person-centred care is, of course, an excellent learning opportunity in itself.

The meaningful evaluation of educational intervention is, however, notoriously difficult to achieve. Our understanding of delirium as an entity and as management practices lacks consistency partly due to the heterogeneous nature of delirium, whereby it presents in a variety of populations with varying clinical presentations and comorbidities. It might be wise to identify a member of staff to take the lead in mandatory delirium training and examining the effects.

All carers, including unpaid family members, need to receive high-quality education, and may even provide high-quality education themselves.

The history of efforts to understand and improve the care of delirium might be framed as occurring in three waves[2] (see Box 13.1).

BOX 13.1 'THREE WAVES' OF DEVELOPING DELIRIUM RESEARCH
First wave
During this first period, delirium was hardly recognised as an important treatment target in routine care.

Second wave

From the late 1980s onwards, there was a marked increase in larger-scale innovation in delirium research. This second wave raised the profile of delirium, stimulating interest in clinicians and policy-makers, and further research efforts continued.

Third wave

The new millennium has seen substantially increased delirium activity on several fronts. New international delirium associations focused on delirium founded in Europe, North America and Australasia, as well as the emergence of several national associations, have catalysed collaborative delirium research.

Possible delirium 'knowledge gaps' in nurses

Nurses are seen as playing a pivotal role in the early recognition of delirium because they spend a substantial amount of time at the bedside and have frequent opportunities to determine the subtle changes in a patient's behaviour that assist in early recognition.

Early recognition of delirium enables prompt diagnosis and management, including rapid implementation of targeted interventions. A reduction in duration and severity of delirium is strongly believed to be crucial as it helps to improve patient outcomes. Conversely, nurses' lack of knowledge and inability to recognise delirium have been previously noted to be problematic in a study of nurses working in a US hospital.

In one study,[3] it was noted that nurses had difficulty recognising delirium, with only 21% able to accurately identify hypoactive delirium superimposed on a pre-existing dementia. Nurses at all levels of experience and education can have knowledge deficits in relation to medication use in delirium and predisposing and precipitating delirium risk factors.

The education of UK trainee physicians

Delirium itself can be introduced in any hospital or care-home induction programme, but the training for junior physicians should go much further than that. The traditional model of 'bedside teaching', involving just medical students and a patient, is flawed in relation to delirium. People with knowledge and skills relevant to a social movement can apply their expertise in positive and useful ways to inspire the call to take delirium more seriously.

The educational challenge in delirium goes way beyond a mere 'spot diagnosis'.

A recent survey of medical schools in the UK reported widespread failure in addressing attitudes on delirium within teaching.[4] This survey revealed that there can be minimal involvement of patients or carers with teaching about delirium, and yet the General Medical Council's 'Tomorrow's Doctors' speaks to a wider need to foster a culture of patient and public involvement, and there is evidence that doing so provides benefits for learners, increasing the likelihood of sustainable changes in attitudes.

Barriers to detecting delirium

At an organisational level, poor leadership, both clinical and strategic, is felt to be an exacerbating factor for lack of prompt detection of delirium. Leaders sometimes hold the view that 'no one will die of delirium', and this is actually factually incorrect. This low strategic and financial priority to diagnosing delirium was seen as a factor preventing improvement in diagnosis, prior to recent attempts at economic analysis. All clinicians who conduct assessments should be able to identify delirium, and it should be noted that this is not just a nursing responsibility.

Barriers to recognition of delirium emerge at both an individual and organisational level. At both levels the lack of immediate recognisable benefit to bringing about delirium recognition was felt to be a major factor to hamper change.

Reasons might include:

- A sense of 'futility' and 'fatalism' – that is, a perceived lack of available interventions even if delirium is recognised (assuming irreversibility of delirium, failure to investigate clinically, and missing potentially reversible delirium precipitating and predisposing factors) – may impede recognition of delirium.

- Ignorance of the theory and practice of delirium, in particular about the benefits of early recognition and treating delirium, emerges as a strong barrier to diagnosis.

- Delirium is perceived merely as a complication of another physical disease and is thereby deemed, inappropriately, to be of secondary importance in itself.

Social movements

Fast progress in improving delirium care will happen because the change is driven by a strong social movement including patients, carers and clinicians.

Delirium education could perhaps include brief education sessions delivered on multiple occasions by 'change champions', supplemented by bedside coaching to improve nurses' competency to assess patients for delirium, and the adoption of resources to support learning.

An important element of the intervention of change is the development of specific measurable outcomes, such as **'ward-specific action plans'**. Furthermore, there has been substantial progress in the use of social media in facilitating learning and discussion of delirium. Contributions are frequently made by established leaders in dementia, and people are encouraged with the hashtag #DeliriumSuperHero. There is even a well-respected Delirium Awareness Day every year.[5]

Interprofessional education

Interprofessional education (IPE) has been defined by the Centre for the Advancement of Interprofessional Education (CAIPE), UK, as occurring when 'two or more professions learn with, from and about each other to improve collaboration and the quality of care'.[6] There are significant benefits inherent in such interdisciplinary research when combined with collaboration with clinical faculty members to ensure the basic science of education research is connected to clinical practice and realises its full potential for patients.

They include:

- Shared purpose and vision, ultimately to create benefits for patients through better educated healthcare professionals, can be achieved by means of a dual focus on how education and training of the healthcare team can produce gain for patients and patients.

- Approaches to teaching where different professions learn together collaboratively are increasingly being encouraged.

- Learning together – where professionals learn with, from and about each other to improve collaborative practice and quality of care.

- The creation of space for the consideration of practice, professional boundaries and reflection around issues of interdependence.

As a corollary, **interprofessional care** refers to 'care provided by a team of healthcare professionals with overlapping expertise and an appreciation for the unique contribution of other team members, as partners in achieving a common goal'.[7]

The effect of education of clinical staff

Studies have identified that education for clinical staff on the detection and treatment of delirium can improve patient outcomes. It is worth noting, however, that merely improving detection rates may not be sufficient in re-orienting a culture of care, because a range of individual and organisational factors which act as barriers to change.

Determining the level of knowledge about delirium can highlight current knowledge needs and facilitate programme development; delirium knowledge can be assessed by interviews and by administering questionnaires/surveys.

Determining clinicians' level of background knowledge is vital in order to design and implement appropriate educational programmes that address delirium.

Distributed leadership

Responsibility for education and training can be distributed across the different levels of clinical nurses and the nurses working with their specific teams, thereby engendering a collective responsibility for nursing staff to engage with the learning. One approach that has been shown to be conducive to learning and improvement in schools is distributed leadership (DL):[8]

> Rather than viewing leadership practice as a product of a leader's knowledge and skill, the distributed perspective defines it as the interactions between people and their situation.

DL is increasingly being studied within healthcare, in a deliberate move away from 'heroic leadership'. DL can be conceived of as a collective social process that involves individuals pooling and sharing their collective expertise such that the overall result is greater than the sum of their individual parts. As more DL progressively emerges and is enabled across the system, cross-boundary and partnership working increases and change happens at a massive scale and pace.

Simulations

Simulations are great fun, and have been found to decrease the anxiety of students in real hospital situations because they can rely on past simulated experiences.

Many healthcare facilities own, or have access to, simulators to educate medical, nursing and allied or associate staff. This is an accepted method to teach nurses about geriatric issues and syndromes, including delirium.

The 'simulation experience' allows participants to synthesise information learned and critically think about the situation.

The simulation session provides time for participant debriefing about the clinical interaction. Participant self-reflection is thought to impact personal professional growth and lifelong learning. This allows learning opportunities in a safe, controlled environment in which no actual patients can be harmed, and enables students to become more proficient in technical skills and critical thinking before they encounter a real patient in a hospital setting.

Grand rounds and the 'patient experience'

Grand rounds within the medical and nursing community have been conducted for many years as a forum to discuss specific cases and appropriate care. They provide an opportunity to link evidence from the literature to clinical practice. The 'recorded' grand round could be later available for online viewing as a preferred method of educational delivery.

Helping families to understand delirium

Helping families understand the risk factors and causes of delirium can assist the entire healthcare team in managing delirium. Primary prevention with significant emphasis on providing non-pharmacological interventions will in future play a strong role in delirium prevention and positive dissemination of education to family members. Informal carers, such as family members, are an important and untapped resource in the management of delirium. One recent educational initiative[9] resulted in the successful development of an evidence-based educational brochure that frontline nurses could use to provide information about delirium to families and to initiate family-driven interventions in the management of delirium.

Web-based learning

Web-based learning provides an alternative approach that helps to overcome the challenges to more traditional educational approaches. It provides opportunities for clinicians to access current information and practice initiatives at a time and place to suit their needs.

Students in academic programmes using web-based learning can tend to perform better than those learning through traditional face-to-face instruction.

E-learning and e-health

E-learning has been identified as an alternative and cost-effective method of delivering education to large groups of hospital staff, and may overcome the limits of traditional educational approaches. It is proposed that its accessibility, availability and use of interactive feedback and real case scenarios make e-learning relatively easier to implement. It is uncertain whether e-learning in itself actually improves patient-care outcomes.

Blended learning, or the integration of face-to-face and online instruction, is widely adopted across higher education.[10] While blended learning is considered more effective than e-learning, blends may not be directly comparable because of the manner in which they are designed.

One vehicle for increasing access to delirium practice tools at the point of care is '**E-health**'. E-Health is the use of information and communication technologies for health. The World Health Assembly in 2018 acknowledged the potential of digital technologies to play a major role in improving public health, where delegates agreed on a resolution on digital health.[11] Over the last decade, there has been a massive progress in E-health, which has led to the creation of multiple online learning platforms for clinicians to stay well informed about the latest treatment algorithms and guidelines.

Further studies might:

- consider approaches to improve adoption and effectiveness of e-learning

- investigate the efficacy of delirium e-learning

- evaluate the extent to which delirium e-learning can actually catalyse behaviour change and delirium practice.

Research is warranted to explore the efficacy of delirium e-learning programmes along with educational initiatives including supporting and empowering strategies.[12]

Endnotes

1   Grealish, L., Todd, J.A., Krug, M. and Teodorczuk. A. (2019) 'Education for delirium prevention: Knowing, meaning and doing.' *Nurse Education in Practice 40*, 102622. Accessed on 2/12/2019 at www.ncbi.nlm.nih.gov/pubmed/31521042.

2   Teodorczuk, A. and MacLullich, A. (2018) 'New waves of delirium understanding.' *International Journal of Geriatric Psychiatry 33*, 11, 1417–1419. Accessed on 2/12/2019 at www.ncbi.nlm.nih.gov/pubmed/29314268.

3   Fick, D.M., Hodo, D.M., Lawrence, F. and Inouye, S.K. (2007) 'Recognizing delirium superimposed on dementia.' *Journal of Gerontological Nursing 33*, 2, 40–49. Accessed on 2/12/2019 at www.ncbi.nlm.nih.gov/pmc/articles/PMC2247368.

4   Fisher, J.M., Gordon, A.L., MacLullich, A.M.J., Tullo, E. *et al.* (2015) 'Towards an understanding of why undergraduate teaching about delirium does not guarantee gold-standard practice – results from a UK national survey.' *Age and Ageing 44*, 1, 166–170. Accessed on 2/12/2019 at https://academic.oup.com/ageing/article/44/1/166/2812362.

5   British Geriatrics Society (2019) 'World Delirium Awareness Day 2019: An opportunity not a problem.' Accessed on 2/12/2019 at www.bgs.org.uk/blog/world-delirium-awareness-day-2019-an-opportunity-not-a-problem.

6   Hosoya, O. (2017) 'Introduction: Interprofessional education (IPE) and pharmaceutical education: Saitama Interprofessional Education Project.' *Yakugaku Zasshi 137*, 7, 847–852. Accessed on 16/12/2019 at www.ncbi.nlm.nih.gov/pubmed/28674299.

7   Heras, G. (2018) 'Interprofessional Care and Teamwork in the ICU.' Humanizando los Cuidados Intensivos. Accessed on 2/12/2019 at https://humanizandoloscuidadosintensivos.com/en/interprofessional-care-and-teamwork-in-the-icu.

8   Spillane, J.P. (2005) 'Distributed leadership.' *The Educational Forum 69*, 2, 143–150. Accessed on 2/12/2019 at www.tandfonline.com/doi/abs/10.1080/00131720508984678.

9   Paulson, C.M., Monroe, T., Mcdougall, G.J. Jr. and Fick, D.M. (2016) 'A family-focused delirium educational initiative with practice and research implications.' *Gerontology and Geriatrics Education 37*, 1, 4–11. Accessed on 2/12/2019 at www.ncbi.nlm.nih.gov/pmc/articles/PMC4708000.

10   See e.g. Bonk, C.J. and Graham, C.R. (2007) *The Handbook of Blended Learning: Global Perspectives, Local Designs.* San Francisco, CA: Pfeiffer.

11   World Health Organization (2019) 'eHealth at WHO.' Accessed on 16/12/2019 at www.who.int/ehealth/about/en.

12   Morandi, A., Pozzi, C., Milisen, K., Hobbelen, H. *et al.* (2019) 'An interdisciplinary statement of scientific societies for the advancement of delirium care across Europe (EDA, EANS, EUGMS, COTEC, IPTOP/WCPT).' *BMC Geriatrics 19*, 253. Accessed on 2/12/2019 at https://bmcgeriatr.biomedcentral.com/articles/10.1186/s12877-019-1264-2.

Afterword

Dr Daniel Davis

This book fulfils its brief in every way – truly the Essentials of Delirium for all who are involved in delirium care. Delirium, the clouding of consciousness, signals a dimming of a fundamental human quality. Dr Rahman addresses this directly by using a deep understanding of the syndrome to frame an approach to delirium care.

Dr Rahman's focus on delirium (to say 'interest in delirium' would not acknowledge how profoundly important he sees delirium care) was born out of a moment of clarity: his first experience of delirium in a loved one. Despite undergraduate and postgraduate study of brain disorders at world-leading institutions, his professional training in delirium had been minimal. Clinical staff didn't have the tools to recognise delirium presentations. No-one was able to explain to him why it was happening and what to expect next.

We are reminded of the power of stories. This story is about someone who had specialist knowledge on frontotemporal dementia, who became a patient in his own right, and is emerging again as a healthcare professional. Truly an expert by experience.

Dr Rahman and I were first in touch on social media. Looking back at those messages from almost two years ago (Twitter DMs end up being a nice record of conversations), we both keenly felt a need to do better on public understanding of delirium and advocacy for delirium patients. We met in real life when he came for a clinical attachment at UCLH – and by then this book was well its way. Later further opportunities arose through our connections at the European Delirium Association conference in Edinburgh. These meetings have a distinct energy and Shibley certainly engaged with clinicians, researchers, policy makers across the board. No doubt the fruits of many of these discussions are embedded throughout the book. We are proud to have him as part of the MRC Unit for Lifelong Health and Ageing at UCL and look forward to continuing our work together.

Dr Daniel Davis, PhD
London, January 2019

Afterword

Dr Amit Arora

Delirium as a medical condition has been known for years; however, it has somehow frequently remained under-recognized, under-diagnosed and under-treated until recently. Delirium is typically a hard subject to tackle but this book handles it brilliantly from start to finish.

This book is intended for the workforce, wherever they are practising in the world, but is equally important for patients, families and carers. It covers both simple and complex issues related to delirium and these all are well explained. Whether readers are interested in emergency presentations, detection, risk factors, differential diagnosis, various measurement scales or post-delirium effects, the book covers them adequately. The book also explains prevention, predictive models and different approaches to dealing with delirium. These are topics which may be of use to all healthcare professionals.

This book should prove useful to all members of multidisciplinary teams in various settings, including the hospital, community and care homes. The book is relevant not only for clinicians, but also for policy-makers and managers. Dr Rahman's passion and understanding of the various aspects of the patient's wellbeing beyond the disease itself is clearly apparent and challenges one to think differently.

In this book, Dr Rahman tells you everything you need to know about delirium, from evidence to practice, policy to law, medication to environment, and from emotion to practical tips of dealing with someone with delirium. Deconditioning, though not a new concept as such, is a recently rejuvenated term and the book addresses this as well, emphasizing the importance of this issue for patients and families. The book also addresses basic nursing aspects such as early mobilization, noise reduction, hydration and nutrition, distraction techniques, communication, etc. He discusses these in the context of person-centred and family-centred care, but also addresses the challenges families and health professionals face when the patient approaches towards their end of life.

This is a book in which patients, their families and friends will also find inspiration and practical assistance. Dr Rahman should be commended for this unique fusion of ideas and practice in the form of an easy-to-read book, which will undoubtedly be found useful by both healthcare workers and the public.

Dr Rahman also touches on the multifaceted approach to delirium care, addressing how to maintain the patient's wellbeing and support the required changes in care as the disease progresses. There are many insights we can take from this book and apply to daily practice.

One of the golden tests of any such medical book is 'Will it change your practice?' This book certainly can do this. Delirium is not an easy topic to address and Dr Rahman must be congratulated for how he has dealt with this. This is a book where science and experience is blended with passion, emotion, knowledge and understanding; and one that not only challenges existing thinking but also provides novel insights and tells us everything we need to know about delirium, in a language that is easy to understand. This, I think, is its greatest contribution to the field.

Dr Amit Arora
Stoke, November 2019

Bibliography

The reader may find the following resources useful as background reading. Further specific references are provided in the main text and are listed alphabetically in the References. The vast majority of the resources below are original peer-reviewed research articles and reviews.

Books, factsheets and guidelines

Page, V.J. and Ely, E.W. (2013) *Delirium in Critical Care (Core Critical Care)*. Cambridge: Cambridge University Press.

Rahman, S. (2015) 'Delirium and Living Well with Dementia.' In *Living Better with Dementia: Good Practice and Innovation for the Future*. London: Jessica Kingsley Publishers.

Rahman, S. (2019) 'A single carer's perspective of dementia.' In D. Truswell (ed.) *Supporting People Living with Dementia in Black, Asian and Minority Ethnic Communities: Key Issues and Strategies for Change*. London: Jessica Kingsley Publishers.

Royal College of Psychiatrists (2019) 'Delirium.' Accessed on 28/11/2019 at www.rcpsych.ac.uk/mental-health/problems-disorders/delirium.

Health Improvement Scotland (2019) *SIGN 157: Risk Reduction and Management of Delirium. A National Clinical Guideline*. Accessed on 28/11/2019 at www.sign.ac.uk/sign-157-delirium.html.

Woodford, H. (2015) 'Delirium.' In *Essential Geriatrics* (3rd edition). London: CRC Press.

Original peer-reviewed papers
Useful preliminary references

Aldecoa, C., Bettelli, G., Bilotta, F., Sanders, R.D. *et al.* (2017) 'European Society of Anaesthesiology evidence-based and consensus-based guideline on postoperative delirium.' *European Journal of Anaesthesiology 34*, 4, 192–214.

Davis, D., Searle, S.D. and Tsui, A. (2019) 'The Scottish Intercollegiate Guidelines Network: Risk reduction and management of delirium.' *Age and Ageing 48*, 4, 485–488.

Bhat, R. and Rockwood, K. (2007) 'Delirium as a disorder of consciousness.' *Journal of Neurology, Neurosurgery, and Psychiatry 78*, 11, 1167–1170.

Inouye, S.K., Westendorp, R.G. and Saczynski, J.S. (2014) 'Delirium in elderly people.' *The Lancet 383*, 9920, 911–922.

Tieges, Z., Evans, J.J., Neufeld, K.J. and MacLullich, A.M.J. (2018) 'The neuropsychology of delirium: Advancing the science of delirium assessment.' *International Journal of Geriatric Psychiatry 33*, 11, 1501–1511.

Types of delirium

Hosker, C. and Ward, D. (2017) 'Hypoactive delirium.' *BMJ 357*, j2047.

Meagher, D. (2009) 'Motor subtypes of delirium: Past, present and future.' *International Review of Psychiatry 21*, 1, 59–73.

Serafim, R.B., Soares, M., Bozza, F.A., Lapa, E. *et al.* (2017) 'Outcomes of subsyndromal delirium in ICU: A systematic review and meta-analysis.' *Critical Care 21*, 1, 179.

Detecting delirium

MacLullich, A.M., Shenkin, S.D., Goodacre, S., Godfrey, M. *et al.* (2019) 'The 4 "A"s test for detecting delirium in acute medical patients: A diagnostic accuracy study.' *Health Technology Assessment 23*, 40, 1–194.

Inouye, S.K., van Dyck, C.H., Alessi, C.A., Balkin, S., Siegal, A.P. and Horwitz, R.I. (1990) 'Clarifying confusion: The confusion assessment method. A new method for detection of delirium.' *Annals of Internal Medicine 113*, 12, 941–948.

Wei, L.A., Fearing, M.A., Sternberg, E.J. and Inouye, S.K. (2008) 'The Confusion Assessment Method: A systematic review of current usage.' *Journal of the American Geriatrics Society 56*, 5, 823–830.

Person-centred care

Clissett, P., Porock, D., Harwood, R.H. and Gladman, J.R. (2013) 'The challenges of achieving person-centred care in acute hospitals: A qualitative study of people with dementia and their families.' *International Journal of Nursing Studies 50*, 11, 1495–1503.

Clegg, A. and Young, J.B. (2011) 'Which medications to avoid in people at risk of delirium: A systematic review.' *Age and Ageing 40*, 1, 23–29.

Dewing, J. and McCormack, B. (2017) 'Tell me, how do you define person-centredness?' *Journal of Clinical Nursing 26*, 17–18, 2509–2510.

Morandi, A., Pozzi, C., Milisen, K., Hobbelen, H. *et al.* (2019) 'An interdisciplinary statement of scientific societies for the advancement of delirium care across Europe.' *BMC Geriatrics 19*, 1, 253.

Prevention and interventions

Bourne, R.S., Tahir, T.A., Borthwick, M. and Sampson, E.L. (2008) 'Drug treatment of delirium: Past, present and future.' *Journal of Psychosomatic Research 65*, 3, 273–282.

Hshieh, T.T., Yue, J., Oh, E., Puelle, M. *et al.* (2015) 'Effectiveness of multicomponent non-pharmacological delirium interventions: A meta-analysis.' *JAMA Internal Medicine 175*, 4, 512–520.

Inouye, S.K., Bogardus, S.T. Jr, Baker, D.I., Leo-Summers, L. and Cooney, L.M. Jr. (2000) 'The Hospital Elder Life Program: A model of care to prevent cognitive and functional decline in older hospitalized patients. Hospital Elder Life Program.' *Journal of the American Geriatrics Society 48*, 12, 1697–1706.

Nikooie, R., Neufeld, K.J., Oh, E.S., Wilson, L.M. *et al.* (2019) 'Antipsychotics for treating delirium in hospitalized adults: A systematic review.' *Annals of Internal Medicine.* doi: 10.7326/M19-1860.

O'Regan, N.A., Fitzgerald, J., Adamis, D., Molloy, D.W., Meagher, D. and Timmons, S. (2018) 'Predictors of delirium development in older medical inpatients: Readily identifiable factors at admission.' *Journal of Alzheimer's Disease 64*, 3, 775–785.

Rubin, F.H., Bellon, J., Bilderback, A., Urda, K. and Inouye, S.K. (2018) 'Effect of the Hospital Elder Life Program on risk of 30-day readmission.' *Journal of the American Geriatrics Society 66*, 1, 145–149.

Delirium and long-term cognitive impairment

Davis, D.H., Muniz-Terrera, G., Keage, H.A., Stephan, B.C. *et al.* Epidemiological Clinicopathological Studies in Europe (EClipSE) Collaborative Members (2017) 'Association of delirium with cognitive decline in late life: A Neuropathologic study of 3 population-based cohort studies.' *JAMA Psychiatry 74*, 3, 244–251.

Fong, T.G., Davis, D., Growdon, M.E., Albuquerque, A. and Inouye, S.K. (2015) 'The interface between delirium and dementia in elderly adults.' *The Lancet Neurology 14*, 8, 823–832.

Jackson, T.A., Gladman, J.R., Harwood, R.H., MacLullich, A.M. *et al.* (2017) 'Challenges and opportunities in understanding dementia and delirium in the acute hospital.' *PLOS Medicine 14*, 3, e1002247.

Palliative care

Hosie, A., Siddiqi, N., Featherstone, I., Johnson, M. *et al.* (2019) 'Inclusion, characteristics and outcomes of people requiring palliative care in studies of non-pharmacological interventions for delirium: A systematic review.' *Palliative Medicine 33*, 8 878–899.

Education

Copeland, C., Fisher, J. and Teodorczuk, A. (2018) 'Development of an international undergraduate curriculum for delirium using a modified delphi process.' *Age and Ageing 47*, 1, 131–137.
Teodorczuk, A., Mukaetova-Ladinska, E., Corbett, S. and Welfare, M. (2013) 'Reconceptualizing models of delirium education: Findings of a Grounded Theory study.' *International Psychogeriatrics 25*, 4, 645–655.

Evidence-based medicine, QI and change

The reader is, above all, strongly encouraged to refer to *How to Read a Paper: The Basics of Evidence-Based Medicine* (5th edition) by Trisha Greenhalgh (Wiley Blackwell/BMJ Books).
Health Foundation (2013) *Quality Improvement Made Simple: What Everyone Should Know about Health Care Quality Improvement*. Accessed on 28/11/2019 at www.health.org.uk/sites/default/files/QualityImprovementMadeSimple.pdf.
NHS England (2018) *The Change Model Guide*. Accessed on 28/11/2019 at www.england.nhs.uk/publication/the-change-model-guide.
Vardy, E.R.L.C. and Thompson, R.E. (2020) 'Quality improvement and delirium.' *Eur Geriatr Med 11*, 33–43. Accessed on 24/02/2020 at https://doi.org/10.1007/s41999-019-00268-z.

References

Adamis, D., Devaney, A., Shanahan, E., McCarthy, G. and Meagher, D. (2015) 'Defining "recovery" for delirium research: A systematic review.' *Age and Ageing 44*, 2, 318–321. Accessed on 29/11/2019 at www.ncbi.nlm.nih.gov/pubmed/25476590.

Age UK (2019) 'Factsheet 62: Deprivation of Liberty Safeguards.' Accessed on 29/11/2019 at www.ageuk.org.uk/globalassets/age-uk/documents/factsheets/fs62_deprivation_of_liberty_safeguards_fcs.pdf.

Age UK (2019) 'Later Life in the United Kingdom 2019.' Accessed on 29/11/2019 at www.ageuk.org.uk/globalassets/age-uk/documents/reports-and-publications/later_life_uk_factsheet.pdf.

Age UK (2019) 'More harm than good.' Accessed on 29/11/2019 at www.ageuk.org.uk/globalassets/age-uk/documents/reports-and-publications/reports-and-briefings/health--wellbeing/medication/190819_more_harm_than_good.pdf.

Al-Aama, T., Brymer, C., Gutmanis, I., Woolmore-Goodwin, S.M., Esbaugh, J. and Dasgupta, M. (2011) 'Melatonin decreases delirium in elderly patients: A randomized, placebo-controlled trial.' *International Journal of Geriatric Psychiatry 26*, 7, 687–694. Accessed on 29/11/2019 at www.ncbi.nlm.nih.gov/pubmed/20845391.

Alagiakrishnan, K. and Wiens, C.A. (2004) 'An approach to drug induced delirium in the elderly.' *Postgraduate Medical Journal 80*, 388–393. Accessed on 29/11/2019 at https://pmj.bmj.com/content/80/945/388.

Alosaimi, F.D., Alghamdi, A., Alsuhaibani, R., Alhammad, G. *et al.* (2018) 'Validation of the Stanford Proxy Test for Delirium (S-PTD) among critical and noncritical patients.' *Journal of Psychosomatic Research 114*, 8–14.

Alzheimer's Disease International (2014) 'Nutrition and dementia: A review of available research.' Accessed on 29/11/2019 at www.alz.co.uk/sites/default/files/pdfs/nutrition-and-dementia.pdf.

Alzheimer's Society (n.d.) 'Deprivation of Liberty Safeguards (DoLS).' Accessed on 29/11/2019 at www.alzheimers.org.uk/get-support/legal-financial/deprivation-liberty-safeguards-dols.

American Psychiatric Association (1987) *Diagnostic and Statistical Manual of Mental Disorders, Third Edition Revised (DSM-III-R)*. Washington, DC: APA.

American Psychiatric Association (1994) *Diagnostic and Statistical Manual of Mental Disorders, Fourth Edition, Text Revision (DMS-IV-TR)*. Washington, DC: APA.

American Psychiatric Association (2013) *Diagnostic and Statistical Manual of Mental Disorders, Fifth Edition (DSM-5)*. Washington, DC: APA.

Andrade, C. (2019) 'Anticholinergic drug exposure and the risk of dementia: There is modest evidence for an association but not for causality.' *Journal of Clinical Psychiatry 80*, 4. Accessed on 29/11/2019 at www.ncbi.nlm.nih.gov/pubmed/31390497.

Antunes, M., Norton, V., Moreira, J.F., Moreira, A. and Abelha, F. (2013) 'Quality of life in patients with postoperative delirium.' *European Journal of Anaesthesiology 30*, 11. Accessed on 29/11/2019 at https://journals.lww.com/ejanaesthesiology/Fulltext/2013/06001/Quality_of_life_in_patients_with_post-operative.33.aspx.

Armstrong, S.C., Cozza, K.L. and Watanabe, K.S. (1997) 'The misdiagnosis of delirium.' *Psychosomatics 38*, 5, 433–439. Accessed on 29/11/2019 at www.ncbi.nlm.nih.gov/pubmed/9314712.

Australian Commission on Safety and Quality in Health Care (2018) 'Hospital-acquired complications (HACs).' Accessed on 28/11/2019 at www.safetyandquality.gov.au/our-work/indicators/hospital-acquired-complications.

Avelino-Silva, T.J., Campora, F., Curiati, J.A.E. and Jacob-Filho, W. (2018) 'Prognostic effects of delirium motor subtypes in hospitalized older adults: A prospective cohort study.' *PLOS One 13*, 1, e0191092. Accessed on 29/11/2019 at www.ncbi.nlm.nih.gov/pubmed/29381733.

Babine, R., Farrington, S. and Wierman, H.R. (2013) 'HELP© prevent falls by preventing delirium.' *Nursing2013 43*, 5, 18–21. Accessed on 29/11/2019 at https://journals.lww.com/nursing/Fulltext/2013/05000/HELP__prevent_falls_by_preventing_delirium.7.aspx.

Babine, R.L., Hyrkäs, K.E., Hallen, S. and Wierman, H.R. (2018) 'Falls and delirium in an acute care setting: A retrospective chart review before and after an organisation-wide interprofessional education.' *Journal of Clinical Nursing 27*, 7–8, e1429–e1441. Accessed on 29/11/2019 at www.ncbi.nlm.nih.gov/pubmed/29314374.

Balogun, S.A. and Philbrick, J.T. (2014) 'Delirium, a symptom of UTI in the elderly: Fact or fable? A systematic review.' *Canadian Geriatrics Journal 17*, 1, 22–26. Accessed on 29/11/2019 at www.ncbi.nlm.nih.gov/pmc/articles/PMC3940475.

Barts Health NHS Trust (n.d.) 'Think Delirium.' Information card. Accessed on 28/11/2019 at www.dementiaaction.org.uk/assets/0002/1206/Think_Delirium_Cards.pdf.

Bauernfreund, Y., Butler, M., Ragavan, S. and Sampson, E.L. (2018) 'TIME to think about delirium: Improving detection and management on the acute medical unit.' *BMJ Open Quality 7*, e000200. Accessed on 29/11/2019 at https://bmjopenquality.bmj.com/content/7/3/e000200#DC2.

Beavers, K.M., Brinkley, T.E. and Nicklas, B.J. (2010) 'Effect of exercise training on chronic inflammation.' *Clinica Chimica Acta 411*, 11–12, 785–793. Accessed on 29/11/2019 at www.ncbi.nlm.nih.gov/pmc/articles/PMC3629815.

Bell, L.V. (1849) 'On a form of disease resembling some advanced stages of mania and fever, but so contradistinguished from any ordinary observed or described combination of symptoms as to render it probable that it may be overlooked and hitherto unrecorded malady.' *American Journal of Insanity 6*, 2, 97–127.

Bellelli, G., Moresco, R., Panina-Bordignon, P., Arosio, B. *et al.* (2017) 'Is delirium the cognitive harbinger of frailty in older adults? A review about the existing evidence.' *Frontiers in Medicine 4*, 188. Accessed on 29/11/2019 at www.ncbi.nlm.nih.gov/pmc/articles/PMC5682301.

Ben Malek, H., Philippi, N., Botzung, A., Cretin, B. *et al.* (2019) 'Memories defining the self in Alzheimer's disease.' *Memory 27*, 5, 698–704. Accessed on 29/11/2019 at www.ncbi.nlm.nih.gov/pubmed/30526307.

Beresford, P. 'Disability, Distress and New Thinking.' Sage Video Tutorials. Accessed on 29/11/2019 at http://sk.sagepub.com/video/skpromo/9llLu8/disability-distress-and-new-thinking.

Beresford, P. *et al.* (2010) 'Towards a social model of madness and distress? Exploring what service users say.' Joseph Rowntree Foundation. Accessed on 29/11/2019 at www.jrf.org.uk/report/towards-social-model-madness-and-distress-exploring-what-service-users-say.

Berridge, K.C. (2004) 'Motivation concepts in behavioural neuroscience.' *Physiology and Behavior 81*, 179–209. Accessed on 29/11/2019 at https://lsa.umich.edu/psych/research&labs/berridge/publications/Berridge%20Motivation%20concepts%20Physio%20&%20Beh%202004.pdf.

Besedovsky, L., Lange, T. and Born, J. (2012) 'Sleep and immune function.' *Pflugers Archiv: European Journal of Physiology 483*, 1, 121–137. Accessed on 29/11/2019 at www.ncbi.nlm.nih.gov/pmc/articles/PMC3256323.

Blacksher, E. (2008) 'Carrots and sticks to promote healthy behaviors: A policy update.' *Hastings Center Report 38*, 3, 13–16. Accessed on 29/11/2019 at www.ncbi.nlm.nih.gov/pubmed/18581931.

Boland, J.W., Lawlor, P.G. and Bush, S.H. (2019) 'Delirium: non-pharmacological and pharmacological management.' *BMJ Supportive and Palliative Care.* doi: 10.1136/bmjspcare-2019-001966. Accessed on 2/12/2019 at https://spcare.bmj.com/content/early/2019/07/30/bmjspcare-2019-001966.abstract.

Bombard, Y., Baker, G.R., Orlando, E., Fancott, C. *et al.* (2018) 'Engaging patients to improve quality of care: A systematic review.' *Implementation Science 31*, 1, 98. Accessed on 29/11/2019 at www.ncbi.nlm.nih.gov/pubmed/30045735.

Bonk, C.J. and Graham, C.R. (2007) *The Handbook of Blended Learning: Global Perspectives, Local Designs.* San Francisco, CA: Pfeiffer.

Borgstrom, E. (2017) 'Social death.' *QJM: Monthly Journal of the Association of Physicians 110*, 1, 5–7. Accessed on 29/11/2019 at www.ncbi.nlm.nih.gov/pubmed/27770051.

Bowers, L., Brennan, G., Winship, G. and Theodoridou, C. (2009) 'Communication skills for nurses and others spending time with people who are very mentally ill.' Accessed on 29/11/2019 at www.kcl.ac.uk/ioppn/depts/hspr/archive/mhn/projects/Talking.pdf.

Brajtman, S. (2005) 'Terminal restlessness: Perspectives of an interdisciplinary palliative care team.' *International Journal of Palliative Nursing 11*, 4, 172–178. Accessed on 29/11/2019 at www.ncbi.nlm. nih.gov/pubmed/15924033.

Breitbart, W., Gibson, C. and Tremblay, A. (2002) 'The delirium experience: Delirium recall and delirium-related distress in hospitalized patients with cancer, the spouses/caregivers, and their nurses.' *Psychosomatics 43*, 3, 183–194. Accessed on 28/11/2019 at www.ncbi.nlm.nih.gov/pubmed/12075033.

British Geriatrics Society (2019) 'Are "frailty units" and "dementia wards" the anathema of pure person-centred care?' Accessed on 29/11/2019 at www.bgs.org.uk/blog/are-'frailty-units'-and-'dementia-wards'-the-anathema-of-pure-person-centred-care.

British Geriatrics Society (2019) 'World Delirium Awareness Day 2019: An opportunity not a problem.' Accessed on 2/12/2019 at www.bgs.org.uk/blog/world-delirium-awareness-day-2019-an-opportunity-not-a-problem.

Bush, S.H., Leonard, M.M., Agar, M., Spiller, J.A. *et al.* (2014) 'End-of-life delirium: Issues regarding recognition, optimal management, and the role of sedation in the dying phase.' *Journal of Pain and Symptom Management 48*, 2, 215–230. Accessed on 2/12/2019 at www.jpsmjournal.com/article/S0885-3924(14)00288-7/fulltext.

Bush, S.H., Tierney, S. and Lawlor, P.G. (2017) 'Clinical assessment and management of delirium in the palliative care setting.' *Drugs 77*, 15, 1623–1643. Accessed on 2/12/2019 at www.ncbi.nlm.nih.gov/pmc/articles/PMC5613058.

Carbone, M.K. and Gugliucci, M.R. (2015) 'Delirium and the family caregiver: The need for evidence-based education interventions.' *Gerontologist 55*, 3, 345–352. Accessed on 29/11/2019 at www.ncbi.nlm.nih.gov/pubmed/24847844.

Cardona-Morell, M., Kim, J.C.H., Turner, R.M., Anstey, M., Mitchell, I.A. and Hillman, K. (2016) 'Non-beneficial treatments in hospital at the end of life: A systematic review on extent of the problem.' *International Journal for Quality in Health Care 28*, 4, 456–469. Accessed on 1/12/2019 at https://academic.oup.com/intqhc/article/28/4/456/2594949.

Carucci, R. (2019) 'Leading change in a company that's historically bad at it.' *Harvard Business Review*, 6 August. Accessed on 29/11/2019 at https://hbr.org/2019/08/leading-change-in-a-company-thats-historically-bad-at-it.

Catchpole, K. and Russ, S. (2015) 'The problem with checklists.' *BMJ Quality and Safety 24*, 9. Accessed on 2/12/2019 at https://qualitysafety.bmj.com/content/24/9/545.

Centeno, C., Sanz, A. and Bruera, E. (2004) 'Delirium in advanced cancer patients.' *Palliative Medicine 18*, 3, 184–194. Accessed on 2/12/2019 at www.ncbi.nlm.nih.gov/pubmed/15198131.

Centers for Disease Control and Prevention (2018) 'Well-Being Concepts.' Accessed on 28/11/2019 at www.cdc.gov/hrqol/wellbeing.htm.

Chang, B.P. (2019) 'Can hospitalization be hazardous to your health? A nosocomial based stress model for hospitalization.' *General Hospital Psychiatry 60*, September–October, 83–89. Accessed on 28/11/2019 at www.sciencedirect.com/science/article/pii/S0163834319302282.

Chartered Management Institute (2011) 'Setting SMART Objectives Checklist.' Accessed on 2/12/2019 at www.managers.org.uk/~/media/Files/Campus%20CMI/Checklists%20PDP/Setting%20SMART%20objectives.ashx.

Clancy, O., Edginton, T., Casarin, A. and Vizcaychipi, M.P. (2015) 'The psychological and neurocognitive consequences of critical illness: A pragmatic review of current evidence.' *Journal of the Intensive Care Society 16*, 3, 226–233. Accessed on 29/11/2019 at www.ncbi.nlm.nih.gov/pmc/articles/PMC5606436.

Clegg, A. and Young, J.B. (2011) 'Which medications to avoid in people at risk of delirium: A systematic review.' *Age and Ageing 40*, 1, 23–29. Accessed on 29/11/2019 at www.ncbi.nlm.nih.gov/pubmed/21068014.

Clegg, A., Siddiqi, N., Heaven, A., Young, J. and Holt, R. (2014) 'Interventions for preventing delirium in older people in institutional long-term care.' *Cochrane Database of Systematic Reviews 31*, 1, CD009537. Accessed on 29/11/2019 at www.ncbi.nlm.nih.gov/pubmed/24488526.

Cole, M.G., Ciampi, A., Belzile, E. and Zhong, L. (2009) 'Persistent delirium in older hospital patients: A systematic review of frequency and prognosis.' *Age and Ageing 38*, 1, 19–26. Accessed on 28/11/2019 at https://academic.oup.com/ageing/article/38/1/19/41354.

Cole, M.G., McCusker, J., Bailey, R., Bonnycastle, M. *et al.* (2017) 'Partial and no recovery from delirium after hospital discharge predict increased adverse effects.' *Age and Ageing 46*, 1, 90–95. Accessed on 29/11/2019 at https://academic.oup.com/ageing/article/46/1/90/2605678.

College of Paramedics (2013) 'The National Ambulance Mental health group.' Accessed on 1/12/2019 at www.collegeofparamedics.co.uk/news/the-national-ambulance-mental-health-group.

Collier, A., De Bellis, A., Hosie, A., Dadich, A. *et al.* (2019) 'Fundamental care for people with cognitive impairment in a hospital setting: A study combining positive organisational scholarship and video-reflexive ethnography.' *Journal of Clinical Nursing.* Accessed on 29/11/2019 at www.ncbi.nlm.nih.gov/pubmed/31495005.

Cornwell, J., Levenson, R., Sonola, L. and Poteliakhoff, E. (2012) 'Continuity of care for older hospital patients: A call for action.' The King's Fund. Accessed on 29/11/2019 at www.kingsfund.org.uk/sites/default/files/field/field_publication_file/continuity-of-care-for-older-hospital-patients-mar-2012.pdf.

Cortes, O.L., Delgado, S. and Esparza, M. (2019) 'Systematic review and meta-analysis of experimental studies: In-hospital mobilization for patients admitted for medical treatment.' *Journal of Advanced Nursing 75*, 9, 1823–1837. Accessed on 29/11/2019 at www.ncbi.nlm.nih.gov/pubmed/30672011.

Crocker, E., Beggs, T., Hassan, A., Denault, A. *et al.* (2016) 'Long-term effects of postoperative delirium in patients undergoing cardiac operation: A systematic review.' *Annals of Thoracic Surgery 102*, 4, 1391–1399. Accessed on 29/11/2019 at www.ncbi.nlm.nih.gov/pubmed/27344279.

Cuevas-Lara, C., Izquierdo, M., Gutiérrez-Valencia, M., Marin-Epelde, I. *et al.* (2019) 'Effectiveness of occupational therapy interventions in acute geriatric wards: A systematic review.' *Maturitas 127*, 43–50. Accessed on 29/11/2019 at www.ncbi.nlm.nih.gov/pubmed/31351519.

Cunningham, C. (2011) 'Systemic inflammation and delirium: Important co-factors in the progression of dementia.' *Biochemical Society Transactions 39*, 4, 945–953. Accessed on 29/11/2019 at www.ncbi.nlm.nih.gov/pubmed/21787328.

Davis, D., Searle, S.D. and Tsui, A. (2019) 'The Scottish Intercollegiate Guidelines Network: Risk reduction and management of delirium.' *Age and Ageing 48*, 4, 485–488. Accessed on 29/11/2019 at www.ncbi.nlm.nih.gov/pubmed/30927352.

Davis, D.H., Muniz Terrera, G., Keage, H., Rahkonen, T. *et al.* (2012) 'Delirium is a strong risk factor for dementia in the oldest-old: A population-based cohort study.' *Brain: A Journal of Neurology 135*, 9, 2809–2916. Accessed on 29/11/2019 at www.ncbi.nlm.nih.gov/pubmed/22879644.

Davydow, D.S. (2009) 'Symptoms of depression and anxiety after delirium.' *Psychsomatics 50*, 4, 309–316.

Davydow, D.S., Gifford, J.M., Desai, S.V., Needham, D.M. and Bienvenu, O.J. (2008) 'Posttraumatic stress disorder in general intensive care unit survivors: A systematic review.' *General Hospital Psychiatry 30*, 5, 412–434. Accessed on 29/11/2019 at www.ncbi.nlm.nih.gov/pmc/articles/PMC2572638.

de Wolf-Linder, S., Dawkins, M., Wicks, F., Pask, S. *et al.* (2019) 'Which outcome domains are important in palliative care and when? An international expert consensus workshop, using the nominal group technique.' *Palliative Medicine 33*, 8, 1058–1068. Accessed on 2/12/2019 at https://journals.sagepub.com/doi/full/10.1177/0269216319854154.

del Castillo, J., Nicholas, L., Nye, R. and Khan, H. (2017) 'We change the world: What can we learn from global social movements for health?' *Nesta.* Accessed on 2/12/2019 at https://media.nesta.org.uk/documents/we_change_the_world_report.pdf, p.11.

Department of Health and Social Care (2009) 'Reference guide to consent for examination or treatment (second edition).' Accessed on 29/11/2019 at www.gov.uk/government/publications/reference-guide-to-consent-for-examination-or-treatment-second-edition.

Devlin, J.W., Skrobik, Y., Gélinas, C., Needham, D.M. *et al.* (2018) 'Executive summary: Clinical practice guidelines for the prevention and management of pain, agitation/sedation, delirium, immobility, and sleep disruption in adult patients in the ICU.' *Critical Care Medicine 46*, 9, 1532–1548. Accessed on 29/11/2019 at www.ncbi.nlm.nih.gov/pubmed/30113371.

Dharmarajan, K., Swami, S., Gou, R.Y., Jones, R.N. and Inouye, S.K. (2017) 'Pathway from delirium to death: Potential in-hospital mediators of excess mortality.' *Journal of the American Geriatrics Society 65*, 5, 1026–1033. Accessed on 29/11/2019 at www.ncbi.nlm.nih.gov/pubmed/28039852.

DiBattista, A.M., Heinsinger, N.M. and Rebeck, G.W. (2016) 'Alzheimer's disease genetic risk factor APOE-ε4 also affects normal brain function.' *Current Alzheimer Research 13*, 11, 1200–1207. Accessed on 29/11/2019 at www.ncbi.nlm.nih.gov/pmc/articles/PMC5839141.

Ding, Y., Niu, J., Zhang, Y., Liu, W. *et al.* (2018) 'Informant questionnaire on cognitive decline in the elderly (IQCODE) for assessing the severity of dementia in patients with Alzheimer's disease.' *BMC Geriatrics 18*, 136. Accessed on 29/11/2019 at https://bmcgeriatr.biomedcentral.com/articles/10.1186/s12877-018-0837-9.

Diwell, R.A., Davis, D.H., Vickerstaff, V. and Sampson, E.L. (2018) 'Key components of the delirium syndrome and mortality: Greater impact of acute change and disorganised thinking in a prospective cohort study.' *BMC Geriatrics 18*, 24. Accessed on 29/11/2019 at www.ncbi.nlm.nih.gov/pmc/articles/PMC5785815.

Doig, C.J., Page, S.A., McKee, J.L., Moore, E.E. *et al.* (2019) 'Ethical considerations in conducting surgical research in severe complicated intra-abdominal sepsis.' *World Journal of Emergency Surgery 14*, 39. Accessed on 28/11/2019 at https://wjes.biomedcentral.com/articles/10.1186/s13017-019-0259-9.

Dougall, D., Lewis, M. and Ross, S. (2018) *Transformational Change in Health and Care: Reports from the Field.* The King's Fund. Accessed on 2/12/2019 at www.kingsfund.org.uk/publications/transformational-change-health-care.

Drasdo, N. (1977) 'The neural representation of visual space.' *Nature 266*, 5602, 554–556. Accessed on 29/11/2019 www.ncbi.nlm.nih.gov/pubmed/859622.

Drummond, M.J., Dickinson, J.M., Fry, C.S., Walker, D.K. *et al.* (2012) 'Bed rest impairs skeletal muscle amino acid transporter expression, mTORC1 signaling, and protein synthesis in response to essential amino acids in older adults.' *American Journal of Physiology: Endocrinology and Metabolism 302*, 9, E1113–E1133. Accessed on 29/11/2019 at www.ncbi.nlm.nih.gov/pmc/articles/PMC3361979.

Dziobek, I., Rogers, K., Fleck, S. Bahnemann, M. *et al.* (2008) 'Dissociation of cognitive and emotional empathy in adults with Asperger syndrome using the Multifaceted Empathy Test (MET).' *Journal of Autism and Developmental Disorders 38*, 3, 464–473. Accessed on 29/11/2019 at www.ncbi.nlm.nih.gov/pubmed/17990089.

Edge Training (2019) 'Liberty Protection Safeguards (LPS): Jargon Buster.' Accessed on 29/11/2019 at www.edgetraining.org.uk/wp-content/uploads/2019/06/LPS_Jargon_Buster_June_2019.pdf.

Egon Zehnder (2019) 'In conversation with Ed Schein.' Accessed on 29/11/2019 at www.egonzehnder.com/insight/in-conversation-with-ed-schein.

El-Gabalawy, R., Patel, R., Kilborn, K., Blaney, C. *et al.* (2017) 'A Novel Stress-Diathesis Model to Predict Risk of Post-operative Delirium: Implications for Intra-operative Management.' In L. Fernandes and H. Wang (eds) *Mood and Cognition in Old Age.* Frontiers Media. Accessed on 16/12/2019 at https://www.frontiersin.org/articles/10.3389/fnagi.2017.00274/full.

Ellis, G. and Sevdalis, N. (2019) 'Understanding and improving multidisciplinary team working in geriatric medicine.' *Age and Ageing 48*, 4, 498–505. Accessed on 29/11/2019 at https://academic.oup.com/ageing/article/48/4/498/5374432.

Engel, G.L. and Romano, J. (1959) 'Delirium, a syndrome of cerebral insufficiency.' *Journal of Chronic Diseases 9*, 3, 260–277. Accessed on 28/11/2019 at www.ncbi.nlm.nih.gov/pubmed/13631039.

England and Wales Court of Protection Decisions: Royal Borough of Greenwich v CDM [2018] EWCOP 15 (29 June 2018). Accessed on 29/11/2019 at www.bailii.org/ew/cases/EWCOP/2018/15.html.

Evidence-Based Mental Health (2013) 'Review: Limited evidence on effects of haloperidol alone for rapid tranquillisation in psychosis-induced aggression.' *Evidence-Based Mental Health 16*, 47. Accessed on 2/12/2019 at https://ebmh.bmj.com/content/16/2/47.

Farzanegan, B., Elkhatib, T.H.M., Elgazzar, A.E., Moghaddam, K.G. *et al.* (2019) 'Impact of religiosity on delirium severity among critically ill Shi'a Muslims: A prospective multi-center observational study.' *Journal of Religion and Health.* Accessed on 29/11/2019 at https://link.springer.com/article/10.1007/s10943-019-00895-7.

Fazio, S., Pace, D., Flinner, J. and Kallmyer, B. (2018) 'The fundamentals of person-centered care for individuals with dementia.' *The Gerontologist 58*, suppl.1, S10–S19. Accessed on 29/11/2019 at https://academic.oup.com/gerontologist/article/58/suppl_1/S10/4816735#.XXFBSvZqWSk.twitter.

Fick, D.M., Hodo, D.M., Lawrence, F. and Inouye, S.K. (2007) 'Recognizing delirium superimposed on dementia.' *Journal of Gerontological Nursing 33*, 2, 40–49. Accessed on 2/12/2019 at www.ncbi.nlm.nih.gov/pmc/articles/PMC2247368.

Fick, D.M., Steis, M.R., Waller, J.L. and Inouye, S.K. (2013) 'Delirium superimposed on dementia is associated with prolonged length of stay and poor outcomes in hospitalized older adults.' *Journal of Hospital Medicine 8*, 9, 500–505. Accessed on 28/11/2019 at www.ncbi.nlm.nih.gov/pmc/articles/pmid/23955965.

Finucane, A.M., Lugton, J., Kennedy, C. and Spiller, J.A. (2017) 'The experiences of caregivers of patients with delirium, and their role in its management in palliative care settings: An integrative literature review.' *Psycho-Oncology 26*, 3, 291–300. Accessed on 29/11/2019 at www.ncbi.nlm.nih.gov/pmc/articles/PMC5363350.

Fisher, J.M., Gordon, A.L., MacLullich, A.M.,J., Tullo, E. *et al.* (2015) 'Towards an understanding of why undergraduate teaching about delirium does not guarantee gold-standard practice – results from a UK national survey.' *Age and Ageing 44*, 1, 166–170. Accessed on 2/12/2019 at https://academic.oup.com/ageing/article/44/1/166/2812362.

Fong, T.G., Davis, D., Growdon, M.E., Albuquerque, A. and Inouye, S.K. (2015) 'The interface of delirium and dementia in older persons.' *Lancet Neurology 14*, 8, 823–832. Accessed on 29/11/2019 at www.ncbi.nlm.nih.gov/pmc/articles/PMC4535349.

Fong, T.G., Inouye, S.K. and Jones, R.N. (2017) 'Delirium, dementia, and decline.' *JAMA Psychiatry 74*, 3, 212–213. Accessed on 29/11/2019 at https://jamanetwork.com/journals/jamapsychiatry/fullarticle/2598160.

Fong, T.G., Tulebaev, S.R. and Inouye, S.K. (2009) 'Delirium in elderly adults: Diagnosis, prevention and treatment.' *Nature Reviews Neurology 5*, 210–220. Accessed on 29/11/2019 at www.ncbi.nlm.nih.gov/pmc/articles/PMC3065676.

Fong, T.G., Vasunilashorn, S.M., Libermann, T., Marcantonio, E.R. and Inouye, S.K. (2019) 'Delirium and Alzheimer disease: A proposed model for shared pathophysiology.' *International Journal of Geriatric Psychiatry 34*, 6, 781–789. Accessed on 29/11/2019 at www.ncbi.nlm.nih.gov/pubmed/30773695.

Fransen, M.L., Smit, E.G. and Verlegh, P.W.J. (2015) 'Strategies and motives for resistance to persuasion: An integrative framework.' *Frontiers in Psychology 6*, 1201. Accessed on 16/12/2019 at www.ncbi.nlm.nih.gov/pmc/articles/PMC4536373.

Gaete Ortega, D., Papathanassoglou, E. and Norris, C.M. (2019) 'The lived experience of delirium in intensive care unit patients: A meta-ethnography.' *Australian Critical Care*. doi: 10.1016/j.aucc.2019.01.003. Accessed on 28/11/2019 at www.ncbi.nlm.nih.gov/pubmed/30871853.

Garand, L., Lingler, J.H., Conner, K.O. and Dew, M.A. (2009) 'Diagnostic labels, stigma, and participation in research related to dementia and mild cognitive impairment.' *Research in Gerontological Nursing 2*, 2, 112–121. Accessed on 29/11/2019 at www.ncbi.nlm.nih.gov/pmc/articles/PMC2864081.

Garrett, R.M. (2019) 'Reflections on delirium – A patient's perspective.' *Journal of the Intensive Care Society*. Accessed on 29/11/2019 at https://journals.sagepub.com/doi/full/10.1177/1751143719851352.

General Medical Council (2008) 'Consent: Patients and doctors making decisions together.' Accessed on 28/11/2019 at www.gmc-uk.org/-/media/documents/consent---english-0617_pdf-48903482.pdf.

Gianfrancesco, M.A., Tamang, S., Yazdany, J. and Schmajuk, G. (2018) 'Potential biases in machine learning algorithms using electronic health record data.' *JAMA Internal Medicine 178*, 11, 1544–1547. Accessed on 29/11/2019 at www.ncbi.nlm.nih.gov/pubmed/30128552.

Gillis, A. and MacDonald, B. (2005) 'Deconditioning in the hospitalized elderly.' *The Canadian Nurse 101*, 6, 16–20. Accessed on 29/11/2019 at www.ncbi.nlm.nih.gov/pubmed/16121472.

Girard, T.D., Exline, M.C., Carson, S.S., Hough, C.L. *et al.* (2018) 'Haloperidol and ziprasidone for treatment of delirium in critical illness.' *New England Journal of Medicine 379*, 26, 2506–2516. Accessed on 29/11/2019 at www.ncbi.nlm.nih.gov/pubmed/30346242.

Girard, T.D., Jackson, J.C., Pandharipande, P.P., Pun, B.T. *et al.* (2010) 'Delirium as a predictor of long-term cognitive impairment in survivors of critical illness.' *Critical Care Medicine 38*, 7, 1513–1520. Accessed on 29/11/2019 at www.ncbi.nlm.nih.gov/pmc/articles/PMC3688813.

Gold Standards Framework (2015) 'John's Campaign – Dementia.' Accessed on 29/11/2019 at www.goldstandardsframework.org.uk/john-s-campaign-dementia.

Gore, R.L., Vardy, E.R.L.C. and O'Brien, J.T. (2015) 'Delirium and dementia with Lewy bodies: Distinct diagnoses or part of the same spectrum.' *Journal of Neurology, Neurosurgery, and Psychiatry 86*, 50–59. Accessed on 28/11/2019 at https://jnnp.bmj.com/content/86/1/50.

Gosselink, R., Bott, J., Johnson, M., Dean, E. *et al.* (2008) 'Physiotherapy for adult patients with critical illness: Recommendations of the European Respiratory Society and European Society of Intensive Care Medicine Task Force on Physiotherapy for Critically Ill Patients.' *Intensive Care Medicine 34*, 7, 1188–1199. Accessed on 29/11/2019 at https://link.springer.com/article/10.1007%2Fs00134-008-1026-7.

Goto, T., Yoshida, K., Tsugawa, Y., Camargo, C.A., Jr, and Hasegawa K. (2016) 'Infectious disease-related emergency department visits of elderly adults in the United States, 2011–2012.' *Journal of the American Geriatrics Society 64*, 1, 31–36. Accessed on 16/12/2019 at www.ncbi.nlm.nih.gov/pubmed/26696501.

Grealish, L., Chaboyer, W., Mudge, A., Simpson, T. *et al.* (2019) 'Using a general theory of implementation to plan the introduction of delirium prevention in older people in hospital.' *Journal of Nursing Management 27*, 8, 1631–1639. Accessed on 29/11/2019 at www.ncbi.nlm.nih.gov/pubmed/31444812.

Grealish, L., Todd, J.A., Krug, M. and Teodorczuk, A. (2019) 'Education for delirium prevention: Knowing, meaning and doing.' *Nurse Education in Practice 40*, 102622. Accessed on 29/11/2019 at www.ncbi.nlm.nih.gov/pubmed/31521042.

Green, S., Reivonen, S., Rutter, L.-M., Nouzova, E. *et al.* (2018) 'Investigating speech and language impairments in delirium: A preliminary case-control study.' *PLOS One 13*, 11, e0207527. Accessed on 29/11/2019 at www.ncbi.nlm.nih.gov/pmc/articles/PMC6261049.

Grissinger, M. (2014) 'Telling true stories is an ISMP hallmark: Here's why you should tell stories, too…' *Pharmacy and Therapeutics 39*, 10, 658–659. Accessed on 29/11/2019 at www.ncbi.nlm.nih.gov/pmc/articles/PMC4189689.

Grover, S., Ghosh, A. and Ghormode, D. (2015) 'Experience in delirium: Is it distressing?' *Journal of Neuropsychiatry and Clinical Neurosciences 27*, 139–146. Accessed on 28/11/2019 at https://neuro.psychiatryonline.org/doi/pdfplus/10.1176/appi.neuropsych.13110329.

Grover, S., Sahoo, S., Chakrabarti, S. and Avasthi, A. (2019) 'Post-traumatic stress disorder (PTSD) related symptoms following an experience of delirium.' *Journal of Psychosomatic Research 123*, 109725. Accessed on 29/11/2019 at www.ncbi.nlm.nih.gov/pubmed/31376870.

Growdon, M.E., Shorr, R.I. and Inouye, S.K. (2017) 'The tension between promoting mobility and preventing falls in the hospital.' *JAMA Internal Medicine 177*, 6, 759–760. Accessed on 29/11/2019 at www.ncbi.nlm.nih.gov/pmc/articles/PMC5500203.

Gupta, N. (2009) 'Complexities related to Deprivation of Liberty Safeguards and Mental Capacity Act in general hospital settings.' *BMJ 338*, b1888. Accessed on 2/12/2019 at www.bmj.com/rapid-response/2011/11/02/complexities-related-deprivation-liberty-safeguards-and-mental-capacity-ac.

Guttormson, J.L., Chian, L., Tracy, M.F., Hetland, B. and Mandrekar, J. (2019) 'Nurses' attitudes and practices related to sedation: A national survey.' *American Journal of Critical Care 28*, 4, 255–263. Accessed on 29/11/2019 at www.ncbi.nlm.nih.gov/pubmed/31263007.

Handley, M.A., Gorukanti, A. and Cattamanchi, A. (2015) 'Strategies for implementing implementation science: A methodological overview.' *Emergency Medicine Journal 33*, 9. Accessed on 29/11/2019 at https://emj.bmj.com/content/33/9/660.

Hardy, S.E. and Gill, T.M. (2004) 'Recovery from disability among community-dwelling older persons.' *JAMA 291*, 13, 1596–1602. Accessed on 29/11/2019 at www.ncbi.nlm.nih.gov/pubmed/15069047.

Hardy, S.E., Dubin, J.A., Holford, T.R. and Gill, T.M. (2005) 'Transitions between states of disability and independence among older persons.' *American Journal of Epidemiology 161*, 6, 575–584. Accessed on 29/11/2019 at https://academic.oup.com/aje/article/161/6/575/80933CARE.

Haugh, J., O Flatharta, T., Griffin, T.P. and O'Keeffe, S.T. (2014) 'High frequency of potential entrapment gaps in beds in an acute hospital.' *Age and Ageing 43*, 6, 862–865. Accessed on 2/12/2019 at www.ncbi.nlm.nih.gov/pubmed/25012157.

Hayden, E.Y., Putman, J., Nunez, S., Shin, W.S. *et al.* (2019) 'Ischemic axonal injury up-regulates MARK4 in cortical neurons and primes tau phosphorylation and aggregation.' *Acta Neuropathologica Communications 7*, 1, 135. Accessed on 29/11/2019 at www.ncbi.nlm.nih.gov/pubmed/31429800.

Hayden, K.M., Inouye, S.K., Cunningham, C., Jones, R.N. *et al.* (2018) 'Reduce the burden of dementia now.' *Alzheimer's and Dementia 14*, 7, 845–847. Accessed on 29/11/2019 at www.ncbi.nlm.nih.gov/pubmed/29959910.

Health Foundation (2011) 'Evidence: What's leadership got to do with it? Exploring links between quality improvement and leadership in the NHS. Accessed on 2/12/2019 at www.health.org.uk/sites/default/files/WhatsLeadershipGotToDoWithIt.pdf.

Health Improvement Scotland (2013) 'Think Delirium: Staff, patients and families experiences of giving and receiving care during an episode of delirium in an acute hospital care setting.' Accessed on 29/11/2019 at www.kingsfund.org.uk/sites/default/files/media/Healthcare%20Improvement%20Scotland,%20Improving%20Older%20People's%20Acute%20Care%20in%20NHS%20Scotland%20-%20staff%20report.pdf

Health Improvement Scotland (2019) *SIGN 157: Risk Reduction and Management of Delirium. A National Clinical Guideline.* Accessed on 28/11/2019 at www.sign.ac.uk/assets/sign157.pdf.

Heras, G. (2018) 'Interprofessional Care and Teamwork in the ICU.' *Humanizando los Cuidados Intensivos.* Accessed on 2/12/2019 at https://humanizandoloscuidadosintensivos.com/en/interprofessional-care-and-teamwork-in-the-icu.

Herzig, S.J., LaSalvia, M.T., Naidus, E., Rothberg, M.B. *et al.* (2017) 'Antipsychotics and the risk of aspiration pneumonia in individuals hospitalized for nonpsychiatric conditions: A cohort study.' *Journal of the American Geriatrics Society 65*, 12, 2580–2586. Accessed on 29/11/2019 at www.ncbi.nlm.nih.gov/pubmed/29095482.

Hodes, J.F., Oakley, C.I., O'Keefe, J.H., Lu, P. *et al.* (2019) 'Alzheimer's "prevention" vs. "risk reduction": Transcending semantics for clinical practice.' *Frontiers in Neurology 9*, 1179. Accessed on 29/11/2019 at www.frontiersin.org/articles/10.3389/fneur.2018.01179/full.

Holly, C. (2019) 'Primary prevention to maintain cognition and prevent acute delirium following orthopaedic surgery.' *Orthopaedic Nursing 38*, 4, 244–250. Accessed on 16/12/2019 at https://journals.lww.com/orthopaedicnursing/Abstract/2019/07000/Primary_Prevention_to_Maintain_Cognition_and.6.aspx.

Holroyd, J.M., Abelseth, G.A., Khandwala, F., Silvius, J.L. *et al.* (2010) 'A pragmatic study exploring the prevention of delirium among hospitalized older hip fracture patients: Applying evidence to routine clinical practice using clinical decision support.' *Implementation Science.* Accessed on 29/11/2019 at https://implementationscience.biomedcentral.com/articles/10.1186/1748-5908-5-81.

Hong, N. and Park, J.-Y. (2018) 'The motoric types of delirium and estimated blood loss during perioperative period in orthopedic elderly patients.' *BioMed Research International,* 9812041. Accessed on 29/11/2019 at www.ncbi.nlm.nih.gov/pmc/articles/PMC6236653.

Hosie, A., Lobb, E., Agar, M., Davidson, P.M. and Phillips, J. (2014) 'Identifying the barriers and enablers to palliative care nurses' recognition and assessment of delirium symptoms: A qualitative study.' *Journal of Pain and Symptom Management 48,* 5, 815–830. Accessed on 2/12/2019 at www.ncbi.nlm.nih.gov/pubmed/24726761.

Hosie, A., Siddiqi, N., Featherstone, I., Johnson, M. *et al.* (2019) 'Inclusion, characteristics and outcomes of people requiring palliative care in studies of non-pharmacological interventions for delirium.' *Palliative Medicine 33,* 8, 878–899. Accessed on 2/12/2019 at https://journals.sagepub.com/doi/full/10.1177/0269216319853487.

Hosoya, O. (2017) 'Introduction: Interprofessional education (IPE) and pharmaceutical education: Saitama Interprofessional Education Project.' *Yakugaku Zasshi 137,* 7, 847–852. Accessed on 16/12/2019 at www.ncbi.nlm.nih.gov/pubmed/28674299.

Hospice UK (2019) 'Facts and figures: About hospice care.' Accessed on 2/12/2019 at www.hospiceuk.org/about-hospice-care/media-centre/facts-and-figures.

Hospice UK (2019) 'What we do.' Accessed on 2/12/2019 at www.hospiceuk.org/about-us/what-we-do.

Hospital Elder Life Program (2019) 'What you can do if your family member is delirious.' Accessed on 29/11/2019 at www.hospitalelderlifeprogram.org/for-family-members/what-you-can-do.

House of Commons and House of Lords Joint Committee on Human Rights (2018) 'The Right to Freedom and Safety: Reform of the Deprivation of Liberty Safeguards.' Accessed on 29/11/2019 at https://publications.parliament.uk/pa/jt201719/jtselect/jtrights/890/890.pdf.

Howard, R.J. (2016) 'Disentangling the treatment of agitation in Alzheimer's disease.' *American Journal of Psychiatry 173,* 5, 441–443. Accessed on 29/11/2019 at https://ajp.psychiatryonline.org/doi/full/10.1176/appi.ajp.2016.16010083?url_ver=Z39.88-2003&rfr_id=ori:rid:crossref.org&rfr_dat=cr_pub%3dpubmed.

Hshieh, T.T., Fong, T.G., Marcantonio, E.R. and Inouye, S.K. (2008) 'Cholinergic deficiency hypothesis in delirium: A synthesis of current evidence.' *Journals of Gerontology. Series A, Biological Sciences and Medical Sciences 63,* 7, 764–772. Accessed on 29/11/2019 at www.ncbi.nlm.nih.gov/pmc/articles/PMC2917793.

Hshieh, T.T., Yang, T., Gartaganis, S.L., Yue, J. and Inouye, S.K. (2018) 'Hospital Elder Life Program: Systematic review and meta-analysis of effectiveness.' *American Journal of Geriatric Psychiatry 26,* 10, 1015–1033. Accessed on 29/11/2019 at www.ncbi.nlm.nih.gov/pubmed/30076080.

Hshieh, T.T., Yue, J., Oh, E., Puelle, M. *et al.* (2015) 'Effectiveness of multicomponent nonpharmacological delirium interventions, a meta-analysis.' *JAMA Internal Medicine 175,* 4, 512–520. Accessed on 29/11/2019 at www.ncbi.nlm.nih.gov/pmc/articles/PMC4388802.

Hui, D. (2015) 'Prognostication of survival in patients with advanced cancer: Predicting the unpredictable.' *Cancer Control 22,* 4, 489–497. Accessed on 2/12/2019 at www.ncbi.nlm.nih.gov/pubmed/26678976.

Hui, D. (2019) 'Delirium in the palliative care setting: "Sorting" out the confusion.' *Palliative Medicine.* Accessed on 2/12/2019 at https://journals.sagepub.com/doi/10.1177/0269216319861896.

Hui, D., Nooruddin, Z., Didwaniya, N., Dev, R. *et al.* (2013) 'Concepts and definitions for "actively dying", "end of life", "terminally ill", "terminal care", and "transition of care": A systematic review.' *Journal of Pain and Symptom Management 47,* 1, 77–89. Accessed on 2/12/2019 at www.ncbi.nlm.nih.gov/pmc/articles/PMC3870193.

Inouye, S.K. (2006) 'Delirium in older persons.' *New England Journal of Medicine 354,* 11, 1157–1165. Accessed on 28/11/2019 at www.ncbi.nlm.nih.gov/pubmed/16540616.

Inouye, S.K. (2014) *The CAM-S Training Manual and Coding Guide.* Boston, MA: Hospital Elder Life Program. Accessed on 16/12/2019 at http://www.hospitalelderlifeprogram.org/uploads/disclaimers/CAM-S_Training_Manual.pdf.

Inouye, S.K. (2018) 'Delirium – A framework to improve acute care for older persons.' *Journal of the American Geriatrics Society 66,* 3, 446–451. Accessed on 28/11/2019 at www.ncbi.nlm.nih.gov/pubmed/29473940

Inouye, S.K. and Charpentier, P.A. (1996) 'Precipitating factors for delirium in hospitalized elderly persons. Predictive model and interrelationship with baseline vulnerability.' *JAMA* 275, 11, 852–857. Accessed 17/02/2020 at https://www.ncbi.nlm.nih.gov/pubmed/8596223

Inouye, S.K., Bogardus, S.T. Jr, Charpentier, P.A., Leo-Summers, L. *et al.* (1999) 'A multi-component intervention to prevent delirium in hospitalized older patients.' *New England Journal of Medicine* 340, 9, 669–676. Accessed on 29/11/2019 at www.ncbi.nlm.nih.gov/pubmed/10053175.

Inouye, S.K., Marcantonio, E.R., Kosar, C.M., Tommet, D. *et al.* (2016) 'The short- and long-term relationship between delirium and cognitive trajectory in older surgical patients.' *Alzheimer's and Dementia* 12, 7, 766–775. Accessed on 29/11/2019 at www.ncbi.nlm.nih.gov/pmc/articles/PMC4947419

Inouye, S.K., van Dyck, C.H., Alessi, C.A., Balkin, S., Siegal, A.P. and Horwitz, R.I. (1990) 'Clarifying confusion: The Confusion Assessment Method. A new method for detection of delirium.' *Annals of Internal Medicine* 113, 12, 941–948. Accessed on 29/11/2019 at www.ncbi.nlm.nih.gov/pubmed/2240918.

Institute for Healthcare Improvement (2019) 'How to improve.' Accessed on 2/12/2019 at www.ihi.org/resources/Pages/HowtoImprove/default.aspx.

Institute of Medicine (1990) *Crossing the Quality Chasm: A New Health System for the 21st Century.* Washington, DC: National Academy Press.

Isaia, G., Astengo, M.A., Tibaldi, V., Zanocchi, M. (2009) 'Delirium in elderly home-treated patients: A prospective study with 6-month follow-up.' *Age (Dordrecht)* 31, 2, 109–117. Accessed on 29/11/2019 at www.ncbi.nlm.nih.gov/pmc/articles/PMC2693729.

Isberner, M.-B., Richter, T., Schreiner, C., Eisenbach, Y., Sommer, C., and Appel, M., (2018) 'Empowering stories: Transportation into narratives with strong protagonists increases self-related control beliefs.' *Discourse Processes* 56, 8, 575–598. Accessed on 16/12/2019 at www.tandfonline.com/doi/full/10.108 0/0163853X.2018.1526032.

Jackson, T.A., Gladman, J.R.F., Harwood, R.H., MacLullich, A.M.J. *et al.* (2017) 'Challenges and opportunities in understanding dementia and delirium in the acute hospital.' *PLOS Medicine* 14, 3, e1002247. Accessed on 29/11/2019 at https://journals.plos.org/plosmedicine/article?id=10.1371/journal.pmed.1002247

Janssen, T.L., Alberts, A.R., Hooft, L., Mattace-Raso, F.U.S., Mosk, C.A. and van der Laan, L. (2019) 'Prevention of postoperative delirium in elderly patients planned for elective surgery: Systematic review and meta-analysis.' *Clinical Interventions in Aging* 14, 1095–1117. Accessed on 29/11/2019 at www.ncbi. nlm.nih.gov/pmc/articles/PMC6590846.

Johnson, M.H. (2001) 'Assessing confused patients.' *Journal of Neurology, Neurosurgery and Psychiatry* 71, i7–i12. Accessed on 29/11/2019 at https://jnnp.bmj.com/content/71/suppl_1/i7.

Jones, R.N., Fong, T.G., Metzger, E., Tulebaev, S. *et al.* (2010) 'Aging, brain disease, and reserve: Implications for delirium.' *American Journal of Geriatric Psychiatry* 18, 2, 117–127. Accessed on 15/01/2020 at www. ncbi.nlm.nih.gov/pmc/articles/PMC2848522.

Judgment: *P (by his litigation friend the Official Solicitor) (Appellant) v Cheshire West and Chester Council and another (Respondents); P and Q (by their litigation friend the Official Solicitor) (Appellants) v Surrey County Council (Respondent).* Accessed on 29/11/2019 at www.supremecourt.uk/cases/docs/uksc-2012-0068-judgment.pdf.

Kahneman, D. (2012) 'Of 2 minds: How fast and slow thinking shape perception and choice (excerpt).' *Scientific American.* Accessed on 16/12/2019 at www.scientificamerican.com/article/kahneman-excerpt-thinking-fast-and-slow.

Kambil, A. (2019) 'Catalyzing organizational culture change.' *Deloitte Insights.* Accessed on 29/11/2019 at www2.deloitte.com/insights/us/en/focus/executive-transitions/organizational-culture-change.html.

Kehler, D.S., Theou, O. and Rockwood, K. (2019) 'Bed rest and accelerated aging in relation to the musculoskeletal and cardiovascular systems and frailty biomarkers: A review.' *Experimental Gerontology* 126, 110643. Accessed on 29/11/2019 at www.sciencedirect.com/science/article/pii/ S0531556519302062?via%3Dihub.

Kennedy, D.B. and Savard, D.M. (2017) 'Delayed in-custody death involving excited delirium.' *Journal of Correctional Health Care* 24, 1, 43–51. Accessed on 2/12/2019 at https://journals.sagepub.com/doi/ full/10.1177/1078345817726085

Kenyon-Smith, T., Nguyen, E., Oberai, T. and Jarsma, R. (2019) 'Early mobilization post–hip fracture surgery.' *Geriatric Orthopaedic Surgery and Rehabilitation* 10, 2151459319826431. Accessed on 29/11/2019 at www.ncbi.nlm.nih.gov/pmc/articles/PMC6454638.

Khan, B.A., Zawahiri, M., Campbell, N.L. and Boustani, M.A. (2013) 'Biomarkers for delirium – A review.' *Journal of the American Geriatrics Society* 59, 2, S256–S261. Accessed on 28/11/2019 at www.ncbi.nlm. nih.gov/pmc/articles/PMC3694326.

Khan, W. (2019) 'An audit cycle demonstrating improvement in delirium diagnosis, prevention and management (NICE) guideline) at a district general hospital.' *Future Healthcare Journal 6*, suppl.1, 14. Accessed on 2/12/2019 at www.ncbi.nlm.nih.gov/pubmed/31363539.

Khoo, S.B. (2011) 'Acute grief with delirium in an elderly: Holistic care.' *Malaysian Family Physician 6*, 2–3, 51–57. Accessed on 29/11/2019 at www.ncbi.nlm.nih.gov/pmc/articles/PMC4170417.

Kiely, D.K., Marcantonio, E.R., Inouye, S.K., Shaffer, M.L. *et al.* (2009) 'Persistent delirium predicts increased mortality.' *Journal of the American Geriatrics Society 57*, 1, 55–61. Accessed on 28/11/2019 at www.ncbi.nlm.nih.gov/pmc/articles/PMC2744464.

Kim, S.Y., Kim, S.W., Kim, J.M. and Shin, I.S. (2015) 'Differential associations between delirium and mortality according to delirium subtype and age: A prospective cohort study.' *Psychosomatic Medicine 77*, 8, 903–910. Accessed on 2/12/2019 at www.ncbi.nlm.nih.gov/pubmed/26397939

Kishi, Y., Kato, M., Okuyama, T., Hosaka, T. *et al.* (2007) 'Delirium: Patient characteristics that predict a missed diagnosis at psychiatric consultation.' *General Hospital Psychiatry 29*, 5, 442–445. Accessed on 29/11/2019 at www.ncbi.nlm.nih.gov/pubmed/17888812.

Koren, M.J. (2010) 'Person-centered care for nursing home residents: The culture-change movement.' *Health Affairs 29*, 2, 312–317. Accessed on 29/11/2019 at www.healthaffairs.org/doi/10.1377/hlthaff.2009.0966.

Kosar, C.M., Thomas, K.S., Inouye, S.K. and Mor, V. (2017) 'Delirium during postacute nursing home admission and risk for adverse outcomes.' *Journal of the American Geriatrics Society 65*, 7, 1470–1475. Accessed on 29/11/2019 at www.ncbi.nlm.nih.gov/pmc/articles/PMC5515080.

Kostas, T.R.M., Zimmerman, K.M. and Rudolph, J.L. (2013) 'Improving delirium care: Prevention, monitoring, and assessment.' *Neurohospitalist 3*, 4, 194–202. Accessed on 29/11/2019 at www.ncbi.nlm.nih.gov/pmc/articles/PMC3810833.

Kyziridis, T.C. (2006) 'Post-operative delirium after hip fracture treatment – a review of the current literature.' *GMS Psycho-Social-Medicine 3*, 1. Accessed on 29/11/2019 at www.ncbi.nlm.nih.gov/pmc/articles/PMC2736510.

LaHue, S.C., Douglas, V.C., Kuo, T., Conell, C.A. *et al.* (2019) 'Association between inpatient delirium and hospital readmission in patients ≥ 65 years of age: A retrospective cohort study.' *British Journal of Hospital Medicine 14*, 4, 201–206. Accessed on 29/11/2019 www.ncbi.nlm.nih.gov/pmc/articles/PMC6628723.

Langmore, S.E., Skarupski, K.A., Park, P.S. and Fries, B.E. (2002) 'Predictors of aspiration pneumonia in nursing home residents.' *Dysphagia 17*, 4, 298–307. Accessed on 29/11/2019 at www.ncbi.nlm.nih.gov/pubmed/12355145.

Larsen, R.A. (2019) 'Just a little delirium – A report from the other side.' *Anaesthesiologica Scandinavica 63*, 8, 1095–1096. Accessed on 29/11/2019 at https://onlinelibrary.wiley.com/doi/full/10.1111/aas.13416.

Lawlor, P.G., Davis, D.H.J., Ansari, M., Hosie, A. *et al.* (2014) 'An analytical framework for delirium research in palliative care settings: Integrated epidemiologic, clinician-researcher, and knowledge user perspectives.' *Journal of Pain and Symptom Management 48*, 2, 159–175. Accessed on 2/12/2019 at www.ncbi.nlm.nih.gov/pmc/articles/PMC4128755.

Lee, S.S., Lo, Y. and Verghese, J. (2019) 'Physical activity and risk of postoperative delirium.' *Journal of the American Geriatrics Society 67*, 11, 2260–2266. Accessed on 29/11/2019 at www.ncbi.nlm.nih.gov/pubmed/31368511.

Li, Y., Ma, J., Jin, Y., Li, N. *et al.* (2020) 'Benzodiazepines for treatment of patients with delirium excluding those who are cared for in an intensive care unit.' *Cochrane Database of Systematic Reviews*, 2. Accessed on 11/03/2020 at https://www.cochranelibrary.com/cdsr/doi/10.1002/14651858.CD012670.pub2/pdf/full.

Linane, H., Connolly, F., McVicker, L., Beatty, S. *et al.* (2019) 'Disturbing and distressing: A mixed methods study on the psychological impact of end of life care on junior doctors.' *Irish Journal of Medical Science 188*, 2, 633–639. Accessed on 2/12/2019 at https://link.springer.com/article/10.1007/s11845-018-1885-z.

Lindroth, H., Bratzke, L., Twadell, S., Rowley, P. *et al.* (2018) 'Derivation of a simple postoperative delirium incidence and severity prediction model.' *bioRxiv*. Accessed on 29/11/2019 at www.biorxiv.org/content/10.1101/426148v1.

Linkaitė, G., Riaukam M., Bunevičiūtė, I. and Vosylius, S. (2018) 'Evaluation of PRE-DELIRIC (PREdiction of DELIRium in ICu patients) delirium prediction model for the patients in the intensive care unit.' *Acta Medica Lituanica 25*, 1, 14–22. Accessed on 29/11/2019 at www.ncbi.nlm.nih.gov/pmc/articles/PMC6008005.

Lipowski, Z.J. (1990) *Delirium: Acute Confusional States*. New York, NY: Oxford University Press.

Lockley, S.W. and Foster, R.G. (2012) *Sleep: A Very Short Introduction*. Oxford: Oxford University Press.

Lucke, J.A., de Gelder, J., Blomaard, L.C., Heringhaus, C. *et al.* (2019) 'Vital signs and impaired cognition in older emergency department patients: The APOP study.' *PLOS One 14*, 6, e02185596. Accessed on 29/11/2019 at https://journals.plos.org/plosone/article?id=10.1371/journal.pone.0218596.

MacHaffie, S. (2002) 'Health promotion information: Sources and significance for those with serious and persistent mental illness.' *Archives of Psychiatric Nursing 16*, 6, 263–274. Accessed on 29/11/2019 at www.ncbi.nlm.nih.gov/pubmed/12567374.

MacLullich, A.M., Shenkin, S.D., Goodacre, S., Godfrey, M. *et al.* (2019) 'The 4 "A"s test for detecting delirium in acute medical patients: A diagnostic accuracy study.' *Health Technology Assessment 23*, 40. Accessed on 28/11/2019 at www.journalslibrary.nihr.ac.uk/hta/hta23400/#/abstract.

Magny, E., Le Petitcorps, H., Pociumban, M., Bouksani-Kacher, Z. *et al.* (2018) 'Predisposing and precipitating factors for delirium in community-dwelling older adults admitted to hospital with this condition: A prospective case series.' *PLOS One 13*, 2, e0193034. Accessed on 29/11/2019 at www.ncbi.nlm.nih.gov/pmc/articles/PMC5825033.

Mahanna-Gabrielli, E., Schenning, K.J., Eriksson, L.I., Browndyke, J.N. *et al.* (2019) 'State of the clinical science of perioperative brain health: Report from the American Society of Anesthesiologists Brain Health Initiative Summit 2018.' *British Journal of Anaesthesia 123*, 4, 464–478. Accessed on 29/11/2019 at www.sciencedirect.com/science/article/pii/S0007091219305562.

Maldonado, J.R. (2018) 'Delirium pathophysiology: An updated hypothesis of the etiology of acute brain failure.' *International Journal of Geriatric Psychiatry 33*, 11, 1428–1457. Accessed on 28/11/2019 at www.ncbi.nlm.nih.gov/pubmed/29278283.

Mannix, K. (2017) *With the End in Mind: How to Live and Die Well.* London: William Collins.

Marcantonio, E.R. (2017) 'Delirium in hospitalized older adults.' *New England Journal of Medicine 377*, 15, 1456–1466. Accessed on 28/11/2019 at www.ncbi.nlm.nih.gov/pmc/articles/PMC5706782.

Marcantonio, E.R. (2019) 'Old habits die hard: Antipsychotics for treatment of delirium.' *Annals of Internal Medicine 171*, 7, 516–517. Accessed on 29/11/2019 at https://annals.org/aim/fullarticle/2749505/old-habits-die-hard-antipsychotics-treatment-delirium.

Marcantonio, E.R., Ngo, L.H., O'Connor, M., Jones, R.N. *et al.* (2014) '3D-CAM: Derivation and validation of a 3-minute diagnostic interview for CAM-defined delirium. A cross-sectional diagnostic test study.' *Annals of Internal Medicine 161*, 8, 554–561. Accessed on 29/11/2019 at www.ncbi.nlm.nih.gov/pubmed/25329203.

Marie Curie (2018) 'Improving support for people with delirium and their carers.' Accessed on 2/12/2019 at www.mariecurie.org.uk/blog/support-for-people-with-delirium/183059

Marie Curie (2019) 'Delirium.' Accessed on 2/12/2019 at www.mariecurie.org.uk/professionals/palliative-care-knowledge-zone/symptom-control/delirium.

Marra, A., Ely, E.W., Pandharipande, P.P. and Patel, M.B. (2017) 'The ABCDEF bundle in critical care.' *Critical Care Clinics 33*, 2, 225–243. Accessed on 29/11/2019 at www.ncbi.nlm.nih.gov/pmc/articles/PMC5351776.

Masman, A.D., van Dijk, M., Tibboel, D., Baar, F.P.M. and Mathôt, R.A.A. (2015) 'Medication use during end-of-life care in a palliative care centre.' *International Journal of Clinical Pharmacy 37*, 5, 767–775. Accessed on 2/12/2019 at www.ncbi.nlm.nih.gov/pmc/articles/PMC4594093.

Massimo, L., Munoz, E., Hill, N., Mogle, J. *et al.* (2017) 'Genetic and environmental factors associated with delirium severity in older adults with dementia.' *International Journal of Geriatric Psychiatry 32*, 5, 574–581. Accessed on 28/11/2019 at www.ncbi.nlm.nih.gov/pubmed/27122004.

Matar, E., Shine, J.M., Halliday, G.M. and Lewis, S.J.G. (2019) 'Cognitive fluctuations in Lewy body dementia: Towards a pathophysiological framework.' *Brain: A Journal of Neurology*, awz311. Accessed on 28/11/2019 at https://academic.oup.com/brain/advance-article-abstract/doi/10.1093/brain/awz311/5587662?redirectedFrom=fulltext.

McCoy, T.H. Jr, Hart, K., Pellegrini, A. and Perlis, R.H. (2018) 'Genome-wide association identifies a novel locus for delirium risk.' *Neurobiology of Aging 68*, 160.e9–160.e14. Accessed on 28/11/2019 at www.ncbi.nlm.nih.gov/pmc/articles/PMC5993590.

McCusker, J., Cole, M., Abrahamowicz, M., Primeau, F. and Belzile, E. (2002) 'Delirium predicts 12-month mortality.' *Archives of Internal Medicine 162*, 5, 457–463. Accessed on 29/11/2019 at www.ncbi.nlm.nih.gov/pubmed/11863480

McKeith, I.G., Perry, R.H., Fairbairn, A.F., Jabeen, S. and Perry, E.K. (1992) 'Operational criteria for senile dementia of Lewy body type (SDLT).' *Psychological Medicine 22*, 4, 911–922. Accessed on 28/11/2019 at www.ncbi.nlm.nih.gov/pubmed/1362617.

Meagher, D.J. and Trzpacz, P.T. (2000) 'Motoric subtypes of delirium.' *Seminars in Clinical Neuropsychiatry 5*, 2, 75–85. Accessed on 29/11/2019 at www.ncbi.nlm.nih.gov/pubmed/10837096.

Medical Protection (2015) 'Mental Capacity Act 2005 – Advance decisions.' Accessed on 29/11/2019 at www.medicalprotection.org/uk/articles/advance-decisions.

Mental Capacity Act 2005. Accessed on 29/11/2019 at www.legislation.gov.uk/ukpga/2005/9/contents.

Mental Health Act 1983. Accessed on 29/11/2019 at www.legislation.gov.uk/ukpga/1983/20/contents.

Mental Health Act 2007, Chapter 12. Accessed on 29/11/2019 at www.legislation.gov.uk/ukpga/2007/12/pdfs/ukpga_20070012_en.pdf.

Mesulam, M.M. (2000) 'Attentional Networks, Confusional States and Neglect Syndromes.' In M.M. Mesulam (ed.) *Principles of Behavioural and Cognitive Neurology*. Oxford: Oxford University Press.

Milisen, K., Lemiengre, J., Braes, T. and Foreman, M.D. (2005) 'Multicomponent intervention strategies for managing delirium in hospitalized older people: Systematic review.' *Journal of Advanced Nursing 52*, 1, 79–90. Accessed on 29/11/2019 at www.ncbi.nlm.nih.gov/pubmed/16149984.

Mitchell, G. (2019) 'Undiagnosed delirium is common and difficult to predict among hospitalised patients.' *Evidence-Based Nursing*. doi: 10.1136/ebnurs-2019-103120. Accessed on 28/11/2019 at www.ncbi.nlm.nih.gov/pubmed/31296611.

Moen, R. (2009) 'Foundation and history of the PDSA Cycle.' Accessed on 2/12/2019 at https://deming.org/uploads/paper/PDSA_History_Ron_Moen.pdf.

Morandi, A., Pozzi, C., Milisen, K., Hobbelen, H. *et al.* (2019) 'An interdisciplinary statement of scientific societies for the advancement of delirium care across Europe (EDA, EANS, EUGMS, COTEC, ITPOP/WCPT).' *BMC Geriatrics 19*, 253. Accessed on 28/11/2019 at https://bmcgeriatr.biomedcentral.com/articles/10.1186/s12877-019-1264-2.

Morita, T., Tei, Y. and Inouye, S. (2003) 'Impaired communication capacity and agitated delirium in the final week of terminally ill cancer patients: Prevalence and identification of research focus.' *Journal of Pain and Symptom Management 26*, 3, 827–834. Accessed on 2/12/2019 at www.sciencedirect.com/science/article/pii/S0885392403002872.

Mouncey, P.R., Wade, D., Richards-Belle, A. *et al.* (2019) 'A nurse-led, preventive, psychological intervention to reduce PTSD symptom severity in critically ill patients: The POPPI feasibility study and cluster RCT.' *Health Services and Delivery Research 730*. Accessed on 29/11/2019 at www.ncbi.nlm.nih.gov/books/NBK545672.

Murray, A., Mulkerrin, S. and O'Keeffe, S.T. (2019) 'The perils of "risk feeding".' *Age and Ageing 48*, 4, 478–481. Accessed on 29/11/2019 at https://academic.oup.com/ageing/article-abstract/48/4/478/5423924.

Mutz, J. and Amir-Homayoun, J. (2017) 'Exploring the neural correlates of dream phenomenonology and altered states of consciousness during sleep.' *Neuroscience of Consciousness 2017*, 1, nix009. Accessed on 29/11/2019 at www.ncbi.nlm.nih.gov/pmc/articles/PMC6007136.

National Academies of Sciences (2002) *The Dynamics of Disability: Measuring and Monitoring Disability for Social Security Programs*. Accessed on 29/11/2019 at http://nationalacademies.org/hmd/Reports/2002/The-Dynamics-of-Disability-Measuring-and-Monitoring-Disability-for-Social-Security-Programs.aspx.

National Institute for Health and Care Excellence (2018) 'Dementia: Assessment, management and support for people living with dementia and their carers.' NICE guideline [NG97]. Accessed on 29/11/2019 at www.nice.org.uk/guidance/ng97/chapter/Recommendations.

National Institute for Health and Care Excellence (2019) 'Psychosis and related disorders: Advice of Royal College of Psychiatrists on doses of antipsychotic drugs above BNF upper limit.' Accessed on 16/12/2019 at https://bnf.nice.org.uk/treatment-summary/psychoses-and-related-disorders.html.

National Institute for Healthcare and Excellence (NICE) (2014) 'Delirium in adults: Quality standard.' Accessed on 29/11/2019 at www.nice.org.uk/guidance/qs63/resources/delirium-in-adults-pdf-2098785962437.

National Institute for Healthcare and Excellence (NICE) (2014) 'Delirium in adults: Quality statement 3: Use of antipsychotic medication for people who are distressed.' Accessed on 29/11/2019 at www.nice.org.uk/guidance/qs63/chapter/Quality-statement-3-Use-of-antipsychotic-medication-for-people-who-are-distressed.

National Institute for Health Research (2018) 'Delirium is common among adults receiving palliative care and could be better recognised.' Accessed on 2/12/2019 at https://discover.dc.nihr.ac.uk/content/signal-000677/delirium-recognition-in-palliative-care.

Neufeld, K.J., Needham, D.M., Oh, E.S., Wilson, L.M. *et al.* (2019) 'Antipsychotics for the prevention and treatment of delirium.' *Comparative Effectiveness Review 219*. Accessed on 29/11/2019 at www.ncbi.nlm.nih.gov/pubmed/31509366.

Nguyen, D.N., Huyghens, L., Zhang, H., Schiettecatte, J., Smitz, J. and Vincent, J.-L. (2014) 'Cortisol is an associated-risk factor of brain dysfunction in patients with severe sepsis and septic shock.' *BioMed Research International*, 712742. Accessed on 28/11/2019 at www.ncbi.nlm.nih.gov/pmc/articles/PMC4022165.

NHS (2010) 'Essence of Care 2010.' Accessed on 29/11/2019 at https://assets.publishing.service.gov.uk/government/uploads/system/uploads/attachment_data/file/216691/dh_119978.pdf.

NHS (2010) *The Handbook of Quality and Service Improvement Tools*. Accessed on 2/12/2019 at https://webarchive.nationalarchives.gov.uk/20160805121829/http:/www.nhsiq.nhs.uk/media/2760650/the_handbook_of_quality_and_service_improvement_tools_2010.pdf.

NHS (n.d.) 'Act Now – getting people "Home First".' Accessed on 29/11/2019 at www.england.nhs.uk/wp-content/uploads/2018/12/3-grab-guide-getting-people-home-first-v2.pdf

NHS (n.d.) 'Quick Guide: Discharge to Assess.' Accessed on 29/11/2019 at www.nhs.uk/NHSEngland/keogh-review/Documents/quick-guides/Quick-Guide-discharge-to-access.pdf.

NHS Commissioning Board (2012) *Compassion in Practice: Nursing, Midwifery and Care Staff. Our Vision and Strategy*. Leeds: Department of Health. Accessed on 29/11/2019 at www.england.nhs.uk/wp-content/uploads/2012/12/compassion-in-practice.pdf.

NHS Confederation (2010) *Feeling Better? Improving Patient Experience in Hospital*. Accessed on 29/11/2019 at www.nhsconfed.org/~/media/Confederation/Files/Publications/Documents/Feeling_better_Improving_patient_experience_in_hospital_Report.pdf

NHS England (2018) '70 days to end pyjama paralysis.' Accessed on 29/11/2019 at www.england.nhs.uk/2018/03/70-days-to-end-pyjama-paralysis.

NHS England (n.d.) 'Personalised care and support planning.' Accessed on 29/11/2019 at www.england.nhs.uk/ourwork/patient-participation/patient-centred/planning.

NHS Tayside, in collaboration with Healthcare Improvement Scotland and NHS boards (2018) 'Think Delirium: Information for patient, families and carers.' Accessed 17/02/2020 at https://tinyurl.com/rlbnru3.

NHS University Hospitals Plymouth (2019) 'Intensive care rehabilitation team named regional champion in prestigious award.' Accessed on 29/11/2019 at www.plymouthhospitals.nhs.uk/latest-news/intensive-care-rehabilitation-team-shortlisted-for-prestigious-award--3023.

NICE Quality statement 5: Communication of diagnosis to GPs. Quality standard [QS63] Published date: July 2014. Accessed on 29/11/2019 at www.nice.org.uk/guidance/qs63/chapter/quality-statement-5-communication-of-diagnosis-to-gps.

NIHR Signal (2019) 'Communication problems are top of patients' concerns about hospital care.' Accessed on 29/11/2019 at https://discover.dc.nihr.ac.uk/content/signal-000758/communication-problems-are-top-of-patients-concerns-about-hospital-care.

Nikelski, A., Keller, A., Schumacher-Schönert, F., Dehl, T. *et al.* (2019) 'Supporting elderly people with cognitive impairment during and after hospital stays with intersectoral care management: Study protocol for a randomized controlled trial.' *Trials* 20, 543. Accessed on 29/11/2019 at https://trialsjournal.biomedcentral.com/articles/10.1186/s13063-019-3636-5.

Nikooie, R., Neufeld, K.J., Oh, E.S., Wilson, L.M. *et al.* (2019) 'Antipsychotics for treating delirium in hospitalized adults: A systematic review.' *Annals of Internal Medicine 171*, 7, 485–495. Accessed on 29/11/2019 at https://annals.org/aim/fullarticle/2749495/antipsychotics-treating-delirium-hospitalized-adults-systematic-review.

Nolan, M., Brown, J., Davies, S., Nolan, J. and Keady, J. (2006) *The SENSES Framework: Improving Care for Older People Through a Relationship-Centred Approach*. Sheffield: University of Sheffield.

NSW Agency for Clinical Innovation (2015) 'Change Management Theories and Models – Everett Rogers.' Accessed on 16/12/2019 at www.aci.health.nsw.gov.au/__data/assets/pdf_file/0010/298756/Change_Management_Theories_and_Models_Everett_Rogers.pdf.

O'Dowd, S., Schumacher, J., Burn, D.J., Bonanni, L. *et al.* (2019) 'Fluctuating cognition in the Lewy body dementias.' *Brain 142*, 11, 3338–3350. Accessed on 28/11/2019 at https://academic.oup.com/brain/advance-article/doi/10.1093/brain/awz235/5549757.

O'Malley, G., Leonard, M., Meagher, D. and O'Keeffe, S.T. (2008) 'The delirium experience.' *Journal of Psychosomatic Research 65*, 3, 223–228. Accessed on 29/11/2019 at www.ncbi.nlm.nih.gov/pubmed/18707944.

Page, V. and Casarin, A. (2014) 'Missing link or not, mobilise against delirium.' *Critical Care 18*, 105. Accessed on 29/11/2019 at https://ccforum.biomedcentral.com/articles/10.1186/cc13712.

Paladino, J., Lakin, J.R. and Sanders, J.J. (2019) 'Communication strategies for sharing prognostic information with patients: Beyond survival statistics.' *JAMA 322*, 14, 1345–1346. Accessed on 29/11/2019 at https://jamanetwork.com/journals/jama/fullarticle/2748666.

Parekh, N., Ali, K., Davies, J.G., Stevenson, J.M. *et al.* (2019) 'Medication-related harm in older adults following hospital discharge: Development and validation of a prediction tool.' *BMJ Quality and Safety*. Accessed on 29/11/2019 at https://qualitysafety.bmj.com/content/early/2019/09/16/bmjqs-2019-009587.

Parker, R., Thake, M., Attar, S., Barker, J. and Hubbard, I. (2015) 'Deprivation of liberty: A practical guide.' *GM: Supporting Healthcare Professionals in 50+ Medicine 2*. Accessed on 29/11/2019 at www.gmjournal.co.uk/deprivation-of-liberty-apractical-guide.

Parsons, T., Tregunno, M.J., Joneja, M., Dalgarno, N. and Flynn, L. (2018) 'Using graphic illustrations to uncover how a community of practice can influence the delivery of compassionate healthcare.' *Medical Humanities*. Accessed on 29/11/2019 at https://mh.bmj.com/content/early/2018/09/26/medhum-2018-011508.

Patient Safety Network (2019) 'Patient Safety Primer: Checklists.' Accessed on 2/12/2019 at https://psnet.ahrq.gov/primer/checklists

Paulson, C.M., Monroe, T., Mcdougall, G.J. Jr. and Fick, D.M. (2016) 'A family-focused delirium educational initiative with practice and research implications.' *Gerontology and Geriatrics Education 37*, 1, 4–11. Accessed on 2/12/2019 at www.ncbi.nlm.nih.gov/pmc/articles/PMC4708000.

Perisco, I., Cesari, M., Morandi, A., Haas, J. *et al.* (2018) 'Frailty and delirium in older adults: A systematic review and meta-analysis of the literature.' *Journal of the American Geriatrics Society 66*, 10, 2022–2030. Accessed on 29/11/2019 at www.ncbi.nlm.nih.gov/pubmed/30238970.

Perlis, M., Shaw, P., Cano, G. and Espie, C. (n.d.) 'Models of Insomnia.' Accessed on 29/11/2019 at www.med.upenn.edu/cbti/assets/user-content/documents/ppsmmodelsofinsomnia2011stheditionproof.pdf.

Petty, R.E. and Cacioppo, J.T. (1986) 'The Elaboration Likelihood Model of persuasion.' *Advances in Experimental Social Psychology 19*, 123–205, Accessed on 16.12.2019 at www.sciencedirect.com/science/article/pii/S0065260108602142.

Porteous, A., Dewhurst, F., Gray, W.K., Coulter, P. *et al.* (2016) 'Screening for delirium in specialist palliative care inpatient units: Perceptions and outcomes.' *International Journal of Palliative Nursing 22*, 9, 444–447. Accessed on 2/12/2019 at www.ncbi.nlm.nih.gov/pubmed/27666305.

Porteous, A., Dewhurst, F., Grogan, E., Lowery, L. *et al.* 'How common is delirium in palliative care inpatient units and what is the outcome for these patients?' *BMJ Supportive and Palliative Care 4*, A61. Accessed on 2/12/2019 at https://spcare.bmj.com/content/4/Suppl_1/A61.3.

Pritchard, J.C. and Brighty, A. (2015) 'Caring for older people experiencing agitation.' *Nursing Standard 29*, 30, 49–58. Accessed on 29/11/2019 at www.ncbi.nlm.nih.gov/pubmed/25804179.

Quality Care Commission (2019) 'Regulation 9: Person-centred care.' Accessed on 29/11/2019 at www.cqc.org.uk/guidance-providers/regulations-enforcement/regulation-9-person-centred-care.

Quinlan, N., Marcantonio, E.R., Inouye, S.K., Gill, T.M., Kamholz, B. and Rudolph, J.L. (2011) 'Vulnerability: The crossroads of frailty and delirium.' *Journal of the American Geriatrics Society 59*, Suppl. 2, S262–2268. Accessed on 29/11/2019 at www.ncbi.nlm.nih.gov/pubmed/22091571.

Racine, A.M., D'Aquila, M., Schmitt, E.M, Gallagher, J. *et al.* (2018) 'Delirium burden in patients and family caregivers: Development and testing of new instruments.' *Gerontologist*, doi: 10.1093/geront/gny041. Accessed on 29/11/2019 at www.ncbi.nlm.nih.gov/pubmed/29746694.

Ravi, B., Pincus, D., Choi, S., Jenkinson, R., Wasserstein, D.N. and Redelmeier, D.A. (2019) 'Association of duration of surgery with postoperative delirium among patients receiving hip repair fracture.' *JAMA Network Open 2*, 2, e190111. Accessed on 28/11/2019 at https://jamanetwork.com/journals/jamanetworkopen/fullarticle/2725493.

Reeve, E., Gnjidic, D., Long, J. and Hilmer, S. (2015) 'A systematic review of the emerging definition of "deprescribing" with network analysis: Implications for future research and clinical practice.' *British Journal of Clinical Pharmacology 80*, 6, 1254–1268. Accessed on 29/11/2019 at www.ncbi.nlm.nih.gov/pubmed/27006985.

Rockwood, K., Lindsay, M.K.W. and Davis, D.H. (2019) 'Genetic predisposition and modifiable risks for late-life dementia.' *Nature Medicine 25*, 1331–1332. Accessed on 28/11/2019 at www.nature.com/articles/s41591-019-0575-3.

Rosa, R.G., Falavigna, M., da Silva, D.B., Sganzeria, D. *et al.* (2019) 'Effect of flexible family visitation on delirium among patients in the intensive care unit: The ICU visits randomized clinical trial.' *JAMA 322*, 3, 216–228. Accessed on 29/11/2019 at www.ncbi.nlm.nih.gov/pubmed/31310297.

Rowley-Conwy, G. (2017) 'Critical care nurses' knowledge and practice of delirium assessment.' *British Journal of Nursing 28*, 7. Accessed on 28/11/2019 at www.magonlinelibrary.com/doi/pdf/10.12968/bjon.2017.26.7.412.

Royal College of Physicians (2015) *End of Life Care Audit: Dying in Hospital.* Accessed on 2/12/2019 at www.rcplondon.ac.uk/projects/end-life-care-audit-dying-hospital.

Rycroft-Malone, J., McCormack, B., Hutchinson, A.M., DeCorby, K. *et al.* (2012) 'Realist synthesis: Illustrating the method for implementation research.' *Implementation Science 7*, 33. Accessed on 29/11/2019 at https://implementationscience.biomedcentral.com/articles/10.1186/1748-5908-7-33.

Saunders, R., Seaman, K., Graham, R. and Christiansen, A. (2019) 'The effect of volunteers' care and support on the health outcomes of older adults in acute care: A systematic scoping review.' *Journal of Clinical Nursing 28*, 23–24, 4236–4249. Accessed on 28/11, 2019 at www.ncbi.nlm.nih.gov/pubmed/31429987.

Saxena, S. and Lawley, D. (2009) 'Delirium in the elderly: A clinical review.' *Postgraduate Medical Journal 85*, 1006, 405–413. Accessed on 28/11/2019 at www.ncbi.nlm.nih.gov/pubmed/19633006.

Schur, S., Weixler, D., Gabl, C., Kreye, G. *et al.* (2016) 'Sedation at the end of life – a nation-wide study in palliative care in Austria.' *BMC Palliative Care 15*, 50. Accessed on 2/12/2019 at www.ncbi.nlm.nih.gov/pmc/articles/PMC4868021.

Schweickert, W.D., Pohlman, M.C. Pohlman, A.S., Nigos, C. *et al.* (2009) 'Early physical and occupational therapy in mechanically ventilated, critically ill patients: A randomised controlled trial.' *Lancet 373*, 1874–1882. See: https://endpjparalysis.org.

Serrano-Dueñas, M. (2003) 'Neuroleptic malignant syndrome-like, or–dopaminergic malignant syndrome– due to levodopa therapy withdrawal. Clinical features in 11 patients.' *Parkinsonism & Related Disorders, 9*, 3, 175–817. Accessed on 24/02/2020 at https://doi.org/10.1353/S1353-8020(02)00035-4.

Shenkin, S.D., Fox, C., Godfrey, M., Siddiqi, N. *et al.* (2019) 'Delirium detection in older acute medical inpatients: A multicentre prospective comparative diagnostic tests accuracy study of the 4AT and the confusion assessment method.' *BMC Medicine 17*, 138. Accessed on 28/11/2019 at https://bmcmedicine.biomedcentral.com/articles/10.1186/s12916-019-1367-9.

Shepherd, V., Wood, F., Griffith, R., Sheehan, M. and Hood, K. (2019) 'Protection by exclusion? The (lack of) inclusion in adults who lack capacity to consent to research in clinical trials in the UK.' *Trials 20*, 474. Accessed on 28/11/2019 at https://trialsjournal.biomedcentral.com/articles/10.1186/s13063-019-3603-1.

Shields, L., Henderson, V. and Caslake, R. (2017) 'Comprehensive geriatric assessment for prevention of delirium after hip fracture: A systematic review of randomized controlled trials.' *Journal of the American Geriatrics Society 65*, 7, 1559–1565. Accessed on 29/11/2019 at www.ncbi.nlm.nih.gov/pubmed/28407199.

Siddiqi, N., Harrison, J.K., Clegg, A., Teale, E.A. *et al.* (2016) 'Interventions to prevent delirium in hospitalised patients, not including those on intensive care units.' *Cochrane Library.* Accessed on 29/11/2019 at www.cochrane.org/CD005563/DEMENTIA_interventions-prevent-delirium-hospitalised-patients-not-including-those-intensive-care-units.

Siddiqi, N., House, A.O. and Holmes, J.D. (2006) 'Occurrence and outcome of delirium in medical in-patients: A systematic literature review.' *Age and Ageing 35*, 4, 350–364. Accessed on 28/11/2019 at www.ncbi.nlm.nih.gov/pubmed/16648149.

Siddiqi, N., Young, J., Cheater, F.M. and Harding, R.A. (2008) 'Educating staff working in long-term care about delirium: The Trojan horse for improving quality of care?' *Journal of Psychosomatic Research 65*, 3, 261–266. Accessed on 29/11/2019 at www.ncbi.nlm.nih.gov/pubmed/18707949.

Silver, G., Traube, C., Gerber, L.M., Sun, X. *et al.* (2015) 'Pediatric delirium and associated risk factors: A single-center prospective observational study.' *Pediatric Critical Care Medicine 16*, 4, 303–309. Accessed on 28/11/2019 at www.ncbi.nlm.nih.gov/pmc/articles/PMC5031497.

Slooter, A.J.C., Otte, W.M., Devlin, J.W., Arora, R.C. *et al.* (2020) 'Updated nomenclature of delirium and acute encephalopathy: Statement of ten Societies.' *Intensive Care Med.* Accessed on 24/02/2020 at https://doi.org/10.1007/s00134-019-05907-4.

Smith, J. and Adcock, L. (2011) 'The recognition of delirium in hospice inpatient units.' *Palliative Medicine 26*, 3, 283–285. Accessed on 2/12/2019 at https://journals.sagepub.com/doi/full/10.1177/0269216311400932.

Smith, M.-A., Puckrin, R., Lam, P.W., Lamb, M.J., Simor, A.E. and Leis, J.A. (2019) 'Association of increased colony-count threshold for urinary pathogens in hospitalized patients with antimicrobial treatment.' *JAMA Internal Medicine 179*, 7, 990–992. Accessed on 29/11/2019 at https://jamanetwork.com/journals/jamainternalmedicine/fullarticle/2731706.

Social Care Institute for Excellence (2015) 'Making decisions in a person's best interests.' Accessed on 29/11/2019 at www.scie.org.uk/dementia/supporting-people-with-dementia/decisions/best-interest.asp.

Social Care Institute for Excellence (2016) 'Mental Capacity Act 2005 at a glance.' Accessed on 29/11/2019 at www.scie.org.uk/mca/introduction/mental-capacity-act-2005-at-a-glance.

Social Care Institute for Excellence (2017) 'Deprivation of Liberty Safeguards (DoLS) at a glance.' Accessed on 29/11/2019 at www.scie.org.uk/mca/dols/at-a-glance.

Social Care Institute for Excellence (2019) 'Liberty Protection Safeguards (LPS).' Accessed on 29/11/2019 at www.scie.org.uk/mca/dols/practice/lps.

Spillane, J.P. (2005) 'Distributed leadership.' *The Educational Forum* 69, 2, 143–150. Accessed on 2/12/2019 at www.tandfonline.com/doi/abs/10.1080/00131720508984678.

Srivastava, R. (2017) 'Dying at home might sound preferable. But I've seen the reality.' *The Guardian*, 1 May 2017. Accessed on 2/12/2019 at www.theguardian.com/commentisfree/2017/may/01/dying-at-home-terminally-ill-hospital.

Steis, M.R., Evans, L., Hirschmann, K.B., Hanlon, A. *et al.* (2012) 'Screening for delirium using family caregivers: Convergent validity of the Family Confusion Assessment Method and interviewer-rated Confusion Assessment Method.' *Journal of the American Geriatrics Society* 60, 11, 2121–2126. Accessed on 29/11/2019 at www.ncbi.nlm.nih.gov/pubmed/23039310.

Stern, T.A., Celano, C.M., Gross, A.F., Huffman, J.C. (2010) 'The assessment and management of agitation and delirium in the general hospital.' *Primary Care Companion to the Journal of Clinical Psychiatry* 12, 1, PCC.09r00938. Accessed on 2/12/2019 at www.ncbi.nlm.nih.gov/pmc/articles/PMC2882819.

Stern, Y. (2009) 'Cognitive reserve.' *Neuropsychologica* 47, 10, 2015–2028. Accessed on 29/11/2019 at www.ncbi.nlm.nih.gov/pmc/articles/PMC2739591.

Stiller, K. (2013) 'Physiotherapy in intensive care.' *Chest Journal* 144, 3, 825–847. Accessed on 29/11/2019 at https://journal.chestnet.org/article/S0012-3692(13)60598-X/fulltext.

Sun, H., Kimchi, E., Akeju, O., Nagaraj. S.B. *et al.* (2019) 'Automated tracking of level of consciousness and delirium in critical illness using deep learning.' *NPJ Digital Medicine* 2, 89. Accessed on 29/11/2019 at www.ncbi.nlm.nih.gov/pmc/articles/PMC6733797.

Takeuchi, A., Ahern, T.L. and Henderson, S.O. (2011) 'Excited delirium.' *Western Journal of Emergency Medicine* 12, 1, 77–83. Accessed on 16/12/2019 at www.ncbi.nlm.nih.gov/pmc/articles/PMC3088378/#b1-wjem12_1p0077.

Tampi, R.R., Tampi, D.J. and Ghori, A.K. (2016) 'Acetylcholinesterase inhibitors for delirium on older adults.' *American Journal of Alzheimer's Disease and Other Dementias* 31, 4, 305–310. Accessed on 29/11/2019 at www.ncbi.nlm.nih.gov/pubmed/26646113.

Teale, E.A., Munyombwe, T., Schuurmans, M., Siddiqi, N., and Young, J. (2018) 'A prospective study to investigate utility of the Delirium Observational Screening Scale (DOSS) to detect delirium in care home residents.' *Age and Ageing* 47, 1, 56–61. Accessed on 29/11/2019 at http://eprints.whiterose.ac.uk/119038/3/DOSS%20primary%20paper_final%20manuscript_author%20accepted%20version.pdf.

Teodorczuk, A. and Billett, S. (2017) 'Mediating workplace situational pressures: The role of artefacts in promoting effective interprofessional work and learning.' *Focus on Health Professional Education* 18, 3. Accessed on 28/11/2019 at https://fohpe.org/FoHPE/article/view/158.

Teodorczuk, A. and MacLullich, A. (2018) 'New waves of delirium understanding.' International Journal of Geriatric Psychiatry 33, 11, 1417–1419. Accessed on 2/12/2019 at www.ncbi.nlm.nih.gov/pubmed/29314268.

Teodorczuk, A., Mukaetova-Ladinska, E., Corbett, S. and Welfare, M. (2015) 'Deconstructing dementia and delirium hospital practice: Using cultural historical activity theory to inform education approaches.' *Advances in Health Sciences Education: Theory and Practice 20*, 3, 745–764. Accessed on 29/11/2019 at www.ncbi.nlm.nih.gov/pubmed/25354660.

Thomson Reuters Practical Law (2019) 'Safeguarding Vulnerable Groups Act 2006.' Accessed on 1/12/2019 at https://uk.practicallaw.thomsonreuters.com/7-500-6748?transitionType=Default&contextData=(sc.Default)&firstPage=true&bhcp=1.

Tinetti, M.E. and Fried, T. (2004) 'The end of the disease era.' *American Journal of Medicine 116*, 3, 179–185. Accessed on 29/11/2019 at www.amjmed.com/article/S0002-9343(03)00666-1/abstract.

Todd, A., Blackley, S., Burton, J.K., Stott, D.J. *et al.* (2017) 'Reduced level of arousal and increased mortality in adult acute medical admissions: A systematic review and meta-analysis.' *BMC Geriatrics 17*, 1, 283. Accessed on 29/11/2019 at www.ncbi.nlm.nih.gov/pmc/articles/PMC5721682.

Traube, C., Mauer, E.A., Gerber, L.M., Kaur, S. *et al.* (2016) 'Cost associated with pediatric delirium in the intensive care unit.' *Critical Care Medicine 44*, 12, e1175–e1179. Accessed on 28/11/2019 at www.ncbi. nlm.nih.gov/pmc/articles/PMC5592112.

Trepacz, P.T. and Van der Mast, R.C. (2002) 'Pathophysiology of Delirium.' In J. Lindesay, K. Rockwood and A. Macdonald (eds) *Delirium in Old Age.* Oxford: Oxford University Press.

Trzepacz, P.T., Baker, R.W. and Greenhouse, J. (1988) 'A symptom rating scale for delirium.' *Psychiatry Research 23*, 1, 89–97. Accessed on 28/11/2019 at www.sciencedirect.com/science/article/ pii/0165178188900376?via%3Dihub.

Twycross, R. (2019) 'Reflections on palliative sedation.' *Palliative Care 12*, 1178224218823511. Accessed on 2/12/2019 at www.ncbi.nlm.nih.gov/pmc/articles/PMC635016.

Ungarian, J., Rankin, J.A. and Then, K.L. (2019) 'Delirium in the intensive care unit: Is dexmedetomidine effective?' *Critical Care Nurse 39*, 4, e8–e21. Accessed on 29/11/2019 at www.ncbi.nlm.nih.gov/ pubmed/31371374.

Uno, H., Tarara, R., Else, J.G., Suleman, M.A. and Sapolsky, R.M. (1089) 'Hippocampal damage associated with prolonged and fatal stress in primates.' *Journal of Neuroscience 9*, 5, 1705–1711. Accessed on 29/11/2019 at www.jneurosci.org/content/9/5/1705.

van der Cingel, M., Brandsma, L., van Dam, M., van Dorst, M., Verkaart, C. and van der Velde, C. (2016) 'Concepts of person-centred care: A framework analysis of five studies in daily care practice.' International *Practice Development Journal 6*, 2, 6. Accessed on 29/11/2019 at www.fons.org/library/journal/volume6-issue2/article6.

van Montford, S.J.T., van Dellen, E., Stam, C.J., Ahmad, A.H. *et al.* (2019) 'Brain network disintegration as a final common pathway for delirium: A systematic review and qualitative meta-analysis.' *NeuroImage: Clinical 23*, 101809. Accessed on 28/11/2019 at www.ncbi.nlm.nih.gov/pubmed/30981940.

van Munster, B.C., de Rooij, S.E. and Korevaar, J.C. (2009) 'The role of genetics in delirium in the elderly patient.' *Dementia and Geriatric Cognitive Disorders 28*, 3, 187–195. Accessed on 28/11/2019 at www. ncbi.nlm.nih.gov/pubmed/19713702.

van Velthuijsen, E.L., Zwakhalen, S.M.G., Pijpers, E., van de Ven, L.I. *et al.* (2018) 'Effects of a medication review on delirium in older hospitalised patients: A comparative retrospective cohort study.' *Drugs and Aging 35*, 2, 153–161. Accessed on 29/11/2019 at www.ncbi.nlm.nih.gov/pmc/articles/PMC5847150.

van Wissen, K. and Blanchard, D. (2019) 'Anti-psychotics for treatment of delirium in hospitalized non-ICU patients: A Cochrane Review Summary.' *International Journal of Nursing Practice 25*, 4, e12741. Accessed on 29/11/2019 at https://onlinelibrary.wiley.com/doi/abs/10.1111/ijn.12741.

Veeranki, S.P.K., Hayn, D., Jauk, S., Quehenberger, F. *et al.* (2019) 'An improvised classification model for predicting delirium.' *Studies in Health Technology and Informatics 264*, 1566–1567. Accessed on 29/11/2019 at www.ncbi.nlm.nih.gov/pubmed/31438234.

Verloo, H., Goulet, C., Morin, D. and von Gunten, A. (2016) 'Association between frailty and delirium in older adult patients discharged from hospital.' *Clinical Interventions in Aging 11*, 55–63. Accessed on 29/11/2019 at www.ncbi.nlm.nih.gov/pmc/articles/PMC4723030.

Victoria State Government (n.d.) 'Preventing and treating incontinence.' Accessed on 29/11/2019 at www2. health.vic.gov.au/hospitals-and-health-services/patient-care/older-people/continence/continence-treating.

Walker, M. (2017) *Why We Sleep.* London: Penguin Random House.

Waterfield, K., Kiltie, R., Pickard, J., Karandikhar, U. *et al.* (2017) 'P-28 Staff experiences of delirium in the hospice setting.' *BMJ Supportive and Palliative Care 7*, 1. Accessed on 2/12/2019 at https://spcare.bmj. com/content/7/Suppl_1/A10.2.

Watson, P.L., Ceriana, P. and Fanfulla, F. (2013) 'Delirium: Is sleep important?' *Best Practice and Research Clinical Anaesthesiology 26*, 3, 355–366. Accessed on 29/11/2019 at www.ncbi.nlm.nih.gov/pmc/articles/ PMC3808245.

Wei, L.A., Fearing, M.A., Sternberg, E.J. and Inouye, S.K. (2008) 'The Confusion Assessment Method: A systematic review of current usage.' *Journal of the American Geriatrics Society 56*, 5, 823–830. Accessed on 29/11/2019 at www.ncbi.nlm.nih.gov/pubmed/18384586.

Welch, C. and Jackson, T.A. (2018) 'Can delirium research activity impact on routine delirium recognition? A prospective cohort study.' *BMJ Open 8*, e0123386. Accessed on 29/11/2019 at https://bmjopen.bmj. com/content/8/10/e023386.

Wenrich, M.D., Curtis, J.R. and Shannon, S.E., (2001) 'Communicating with dying patients within the spectrum of medical care from terminal diagnosis to death.' *JAMA Internal Medicine 161*, 6, 868–874. Accessed on 2/12/2019 at https://jamanetwork.com/journals/jamainternalmedicine/fullarticle/647723.

Wetli, C.V. and Fishbain, D.A. (1985) 'Cocaine-induced psychosis and sudden death in recreational cocaine users.' *Journal of Forensic Sciences 30*, 3, 873–80. Accessed on 16/12/2019 at www.ncbi.nlm.nih.gov/pubmed/4031813.

Williams, B. (2019) 'The National Early Warning Score and the acutely confused patient.' *Clinical Medicine 19*, 2, 190–191. Accessed on 16/12/2019 at www.ncbi.nlm.nih.gov/pmc/articles/PMC6454357.

World Federation of Occupational Therapists (2019) 'About Occupational Therapy.' Accessed on 29/11/2019 at www.wfot.org/about-occupational-therapy.

World Health Organization (1992) *The ICD-10 Classification of Mental and Behavioural Disorders: Clinical Descriptions and Diagnostic Guidelines.* Geneva: WHO.

World Health Organization (2007) *Scoping Paper: Priority Public Health Conditions.* Geneva: WHO. Accessed on 13/12/2019 at www.who.int/social_determinants/resources/pphc_scoping_paper.pdf.

World Health Organization (2019) 'WHO Definition of Palliative Care.' Accessed on 2/12/2019 at www.who.int/cancer/palliative/definition/en.

World Health Organization (2019) 'eHealth at WHO.' Accessed on 16/12/2019 at www.who.int/ehealth/about/en.

World Health Organization (n.d.) 'Equity.' Accessed on 2/12/2019 at www.who.int/healthsystems/topics/equity/en.

Yamada, C., Iwawaki, Y., Harada, K., Fukui, M., Morimoto, M. and Yamanaka, R. (2018) 'Frequency and risk factors for subsyndromal delirium in an intensive care unit.' *Intensive and Critical Care Nursing 47*, 15–22. Accessed on 28/11/2019 at www.ncbi.nlm.nih.gov/pubmed/29606481.

Young, J. and Inouye, S.K. (2007) 'Delirium in older people.' *BMJ 334*, 7598, 842–846. Accessed on 16/12/2019 at www.ncbi.nlm.nih.gov/pmc/articles/PMC1853193.

Zeng, H., Li, Z., He, J. and Fu, W. (2019) 'Dexmedetomidine for the prevention of postoperative delirium in elderly patients undergoing noncardiac surgery: A meta-analysis of randomized controlled trials.' *PLOS One.* Accessed on 29/11/2019 at https://journals.plos.org/plosone/article?id=10.1371/journal.pone.0218088.

Zhang, Q., Gao, F., Zhang, S., Sun, W. and Li, Z. (2019) 'Prophylactic use of exogenous melatonin and melatonin receptor agonists to improve sleep and delirium in the intensive care units: A systematic review and meta-analysis of randomized controlled trials.' *Sleep and Breathing 23*, 4, 1059–1070. Accessed on 29/11/2019 at www.ncbi.nlm.nih.gov/pubmed/31119597.

Zipser, C.M., Deuel, J., Ernst, J., Schubert, M. *et al.* (2019) 'Predisposing and precipitating factors for delirium in neurology: A prospective cohort study of 1487 patients.' *Journal of Neurology 266*, 12, 3065–3075. Accessed on 28/11/2019 at www.ncbi.nlm.nih.gov/pubmed/31520105.

Zipser, C.M., Knoepfel, S., Hayoz, P., Schubert, M. *et al.* (2019) 'Clinical management of delirium: The response depends on the subtypes. An observational cohort study in 602 patients.' *Palliative and Supportive Care*, 1–8, doi:10.1017/S1478951519000609. Accessed on 28/11/2019 at www.ncbi.nlm.nih.gov/pubmed/31506133.